DEADLY DISEASES AND EPIDEMICS

ESCHERICHIA COLI
INFECTIONS

DEADLY DISEASES AND EPIDEMICS

DEADLY DISEASES AND EPIDEMICS

ESCHERICHIA COLI
INFECTIONS

Shannon D. Manning

CONSULTING EDITOR
The Late I. Edward Alcamo
The Late Distinguished Teaching Professor of Microbiology,
SUNY Farmingdale

FOREWORD BY
David Heymann
World Health Organization

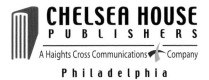

CHELSEA HOUSE
PUBLISHERS
A Haights Cross Communications Company
Philadelphia

Dedication
We dedicate the books in the DEADLY DISEASES AND EPIDEMICS series to Ed Alcamo, whose wit, charm, intelligence, and commitment to biology education were second to none.

Cover: An example of the *Escherichia coli* bacterium that can cause gastrointestinal distress. This photomicrograph was taken with a scanning electron microscope at a magnification of x21,428.

CHELSEA HOUSE PUBLISHERS
VP, NEW PRODUCT DEVELOPMENT Sally Cheney
DIRECTOR OF PRODUCTION Kim Shinners
CREATIVE MANAGER Takeshi Takahashi
MANUFACTURING MANAGER Diann Grasse

Staff for *Escherichia coli* Infections
EXECUTIVE EDITOR Tara Koellhoffer
ASSOCIATE EDITOR Beth Reger
PRODUCTION EDITOR Noelle Nardone
PHOTO EDITOR Sarah Bloom
SERIES DESIGNER Terry Mallon
COVER DESIGNER Keith Trego
LAYOUT 21st Century Publishing and Communications, Inc.

A Haights Cross Communications ✦ Company

http://www.chelseahouse.com

First Printing

1 3 5 7 9 8 6 4 2

Library of Congress Cataloging-in-Publication Data

Manning, Shannon D., 1971-
    Escherichia coli infections / Shannon D. Manning.
        p. cm.—(Deadly diseases and epidemics)
Includes bibliographical references and index.
    ISBN 0-7910-7949-X (hardcover) — ISBN 0-7910-8343-8 (pbk.)
1. Escherichia coli infections. 2. Escherichia coli. I. Title. II. Series.
QR82.E6M36 2004
616.9'26—dc22

                                                    2004012323

Table of Contents

25.95

Foreword

In the 1960s, many of the infectious diseases that had terrorized generations were tamed. After a century of advances, the leading killers of Americans both young and old were being prevented with new vaccines or cured with new medicines. The risk of death from pneumonia, tuberculosis (TB), meningitis, influenza, whooping cough, and diphtheria declined dramatically. New vaccines lifted the fear that summer would bring polio, and a global campaign was on the verge of eradicating smallpox worldwide. New pesticides like DDT cleared mosquitoes from homes and fields, thus reducing the incidence of malaria, which was present in the southern United States and which remains a leading killer of children worldwide. New technologies produced safe drinking water and removed the risk of cholera and other water-borne diseases. Science seemed unstoppable. Disease seemed destined to all but disappear.

But the euphoria of the 1960s has evaporated.

The microbes fought back. Those causing diseases like TB and malaria evolved resistance to cheap and effective drugs. The mosquito developed the ability to defuse pesticides. New diseases emerged, including AIDS, Legionnaires, and Lyme disease. And diseases which had not been seen in decades re-emerged, as the hantavirus did in the Navajo Nation in 1993. Technology itself actually created new health risks. The global transportation network, for example, meant that diseases like West Nile virus could spread beyond isolated regions and quickly become global threats. Even modern public health protections sometimes failed, as they did in 1993 in Milwaukee, Wisconsin, resulting in 400,000 cases of the digestive system illness cryptosporidiosis. And, more recently, the threat from smallpox, a disease believed to be completely eradicated, has returned along with other potential bioterrorism weapons such as anthrax.

The lesson is that the fight against infectious diseases will never end.

In our constant struggle against disease, we as individuals have a weapon that does not require vaccines or drugs, and that is the warehouse of knowledge. We learn from the history of science that "modern" beliefs can be wrong. In this series of books, for example, you will learn that diseases like syphilis were once thought to be caused by eating potatoes. The invention of the microscope set science on the right path. There are more positive lessons from history. For example, smallpox was eliminated by vaccinating everyone who had come in contact with an infected person. This "ring" approach to smallpox control is still the preferred method for confronting an outbreak, should the disease be intentionally reintroduced.

At the same time, we are constantly adding new drugs, new vaccines, and new information to the warehouse. Recently, the entire human genome was decoded. So too was the genome of the parasite that causes malaria. Perhaps by looking at the microbe and the victim through the lens of genetics we will be able to discover new ways to fight malaria, which remains the leading killer of children in many countries.

Because of advances in our understanding of such diseases as AIDS, entire new classes of anti-retroviral drugs have been developed. But resistance to all these drugs has already been detected, so we know that AIDS drug development must continue.

Education, experimentation, and the discoveries that grow out of them are the best tools to protect health. Opening this book may put you on the path of discovery. I hope so, because new vaccines, new antibiotics, new technologies, and, most importantly, new scientists are needed now more than ever if we are to remain on the winning side of this struggle against microbes.

David Heymann
Executive Director
Communicable Diseases Section
World Health Organization
Geneva, Switzerland

1

Tainted Food

In early 1982, approximately 47 healthy adults and children living in Oregon and Michigan developed a severe illness with symptoms of stomach pain and cramping followed by episodes of bloody diarrhea.[1] At first, the cause of this disease was a mystery because all the routine laboratory tests were negative for the known causes of diarrheal illnesses. As a result, no one knew how to treat the sick patients.

The culprit—a type of bacteria called *Escherichia coli* O157:H7—was ultimately found to be responsible for the outbreak of severe diarrhea. This finding was quite a surprise to health-care professionals, because *E. coli* (the name *Escherichia coli* is often shortened to *E. coli* for ease of reference) bacteria are very common and generally exist in people's bodies without causing disease. In addition, this newly identified type (O157:H7) was rare and had previously been implicated in only one other case of bloody diarrhea, back in 1975.[2] The next step was to determine how these patients had acquired such a new and rare infection. A tedious and costly investigation was required to answer this question.

After questioning each patient involved in the outbreak extensively, investigators determined that the victims likely acquired the *E. coli* O157:H7 bacterium through food—specifically, from raw or undercooked hamburgers purchased at certain McDonald's® fast-food restaurants. An inspection of the restaurants revealed that the hamburger meat was not being cooked thoroughly and that the bacteria could therefore survive in the meat and be passed on to people.

IS *E. COLI* O157:H7 REALLY DANGEROUS?
After scientists discovered that meat could be the source for a new infectious

DISEASE DETECTIVES

In 1946, the federal government created an agency called the Communicable Disease Center (CDC) in Atlanta, Georgia. The primary role of this agency was to oversee and support state health agencies in the fight against infectious diseases—diseases caused by an agent, such as a virus, bacterium, or parasite. The Epidemic Intelligence Service (EIS), which consists of medical doctors, researchers, and scientists who investigate all types of infectious disease epidemics, was developed in 1951. The creation of this agency enabled the CDC to broaden its scope. EIS officers are often referred to as "disease detectives," because their job is to determine the cause of disease outbreaks, prevent future infections, and help to promote healthy lifestyles. These objectives are critical for maintaining public health.

In 1992, the CDC was renamed the Centers for Disease Control and Prevention, to reflect its role in the prevention of injuries and all diseases, which includes diseases of a non-infectious origin (such as cancer and diabetes) as well. Today, the CDC is still primarily housed in Atlanta, although it has numerous facilities throughout the nation and in other countries.[a]

In 1948, only two years after the creation of the CDC, another important entity—the World Health Organization (WHO)—was created. The mission of the WHO was similar to that of the CDC; however, the WHO monitors disease throughout the entire world. Information exchange among health-care officials worldwide has become critical to the understanding of the causes and prevention of diseases.

The CDC Mission

"To promote health and quality of life by preventing and controlling disease, injury, and disability."[b]

a. Centers for Disease Control and Prevention. *CDC Timeline, 2001.* Available online at *http://www.cdc.gov/od/oc/media/timeline.htm.*

b. Centers for Disease Control and Prevention. *CDC Mission, 2003.* Available online at *http://www.cdc.gov/aboutcdc.htm#mission.*

disease, everyone started to point fingers. The public blamed the restaurants, the restaurants blamed the meat supplier, the supplier blamed the meat-processing plant, the plant blamed farmers, and so on. No one could decide who was actually to blame and whether the disease was even significant enough to fight over. After all, the outbreak caused no deaths and only made 47 people ill.

However, **sporadic**, random, isolated cases continued to occur. Another McDonald's outbreak occurred in the Midwest in 1984. This one more definitively pointed to meat as the source of the infections. Additionally, four adults living in a Nebraska nursing home died from the illness, along with two adults from the state of Washington. Three children in North Carolina developed a very severe, long-term complication called **hemolytic uremic syndrome** (**HUS**) after the diarrhea had subsided. HUS can cause kidney failure and often leads to death, particularly among children. All nine of these infections were reportedly associated with *E. coli* O157:H7, although the source was unknown.[3]

E. COLI O157:H7 STRIKES AGAIN

In January 1993, *E. coli* O157:H7 returned with a vengeance in Washington, California, Nevada, and Utah, causing one of the nation's most serious food-poisoning outbreaks. The source of the outbreak was hamburgers sold at various Jack in the Box® fast-food restaurants. By April 1993, more than 700 people had developed diarrheal disease symptoms, and 56 of them had developed HUS. Of these, 4 people—all children—died.[4]

Once again, *E. coli* O157:H7 was implicated as the cause of the outbreak, and the specific culprit was the Jack in the Box "Monster Burger." This burger, part of a special promotion, was sold at a reduced price. Ironically, the slogan for the promotion was, "So good it's scary." Demand for the burgers was unusually high, and the restaurant had difficulty keeping up with it. As a result, the burgers were not cooked long enough to kill the *E. coli* bacterium.[5]

Following the chaos associated with the outbreak, most of the victims hired attorneys and the lawsuits began. Jack in the Box sued the meat suppliers, and, in turn, the suppliers sued their suppliers. The largest personal-injury settlement—in the amount of $15.6 million—went to the family of a 9-year-old girl who was in a coma for 42 days after eating a contaminated hamburger. The girl is still suffering from injuries as a result of the infection.[6]

OUTBREAKS OUTSIDE THE UNITED STATES

Many people initially thought that the *E. coli* O157:H7 problem was isolated. This view changed considerably when Sakai City, Japan, was overwhelmed by the largest *E. coli* O157:H7 outbreak to date. Approximately 10,000 people were infected with *E. coli* O157:H7 in the course of a few months; 6,000 of these individuals were children, 12 of whom died. The source of the outbreak was found to be radish sprouts that were included in children's school lunches. Radish sprouts also were associated with another Japanese *E. coli* outbreak in a Kyoto factory a few months later. The outbreak caused diarrheal disease in 74 factory workers, HUS in 3, and the death of one person. Contaminated radish sprouts in lunches sold in the factory cafeteria over a one-week period were the suspected culprit.[7]

Another serious *E. coli* O157:H7 outbreak also occurred during 1996, this one in Lanarkshire, Scotland. Authorities reported 490 cases and 18 deaths; the source of the infection was contaminated meat sold by one butcher.[8]

CONTAMINATION OF NONMEAT SOURCES

Up until the radish sprout outbreak in Japan, contaminated meat products were thought to be the primary cause of *E. coli* O157:H7 infections. Because of this, many government agencies became committed to enhancing the meat inspection process in the United States. Although this has had a positive impact on the number and extent of meat-associated *E. coli* O157:H7 outbreaks, it has not affected incidence of contamination of nonmeat sources.

THE NORTHWESTERN UNITED STATES, 1996

A large multistate *E. coli* outbreak in 1996 gained an unusual amount of attention from the media, public, and health-care workers nationwide. The primary reason for this was because the source of the bacterium was apple juice. Odwalla, a well-known fruit juice manufacturer based in Half Moon Bay, California, processed and bottled unpasteurized, fresh-squeezed apple juice for distribution throughout the Northwest. Pasteurization—a technique that is commonly used to treat milk and other beverages—readily kills bacteria that may be present. If a beverage is unpasteurized, however, the chance of contamination increases significantly. During this outbreak, more than 60 people became ill from *E. coli* O157:H7–associated infections and a 16-month-old child died.[9]

PENNSYLVANIA, 2000

In Montgomery County, Pennsylvania, 51 people fell ill with an *E. coli* O157:H7–associated diarrheal illness that caused HUS in 15 of the victims. Most of the affected patients were school-age children. The Centers for Disease Control and Prevention (CDC) worked with various Pennsylvania health departments to identify the cause of the outbreak. Each patient was given a survey and asked to answer numerous questions about his or her behaviors and diet prior to the onset of the illness.

After tallying the results, investigators identified a school trip to a specific dairy farm as the contaminating event; however, no one knew which part of the farm was contaminated. Investigators used cotton swabs to take samples at different places on the farm, including from the animals, to assess whether the *E. coli* O157:H7 bacterium were present.

Table 1.1 Other notable *E. coli* O157:H7 infections that have been reported to the CDC since 1990

Year	Location	Source of Infection	Number of people affected		
			Diarrhea	HUS	Deaths
1990	North Dakota	Rare roast beef	70	2	0
1994	Montana	Dry-cured salami	20	1	0
1995	Illinois	Swimming in a contaminated lake	12	3	0
1996	Connecticut and New York	Unpasteurized apple cider	8	2	0
1997	Michigan and Virginia	Raw alfalfa sprouts	93	10	0
1998	Alpine, Wyoming	Contaminated water supply	157	4	0
1998	Wisconsin	Fresh cheese curds from a dairy plant	55	0	0
1999	Washington County Fair, New York	Contaminated well water	921	11	2
2000	Washington	Petting zoo	5	1	0
2002	Lane County Fair, Oregon	Sheep and goat expo hall	>75	12	0
2002	Cheerleading camp, Washington	Contaminated lettuce	>29	1	0

In addition to finding *E. coli* O157:H7 on a handrail at the farm, 28 of the 216 cows tested positive; none of the other 43 animal types tested positive for the bacteria. Additionally, the survey results revealed that specific behaviors promoting hand-to-mouth contact, such as biting nails and eating food before handwashing, were more common in infected patients than in the healthy individuals who visited the same farm. Based on this evidence, the investigators concluded that the cows were the **reservoir**, or source, of the infectious agent, and that most patients must have acquired the bacterium by petting the cows. Eating lunch without handwashing would have given the bacterium access to the body, thereby initiating the disease process.

E. COLI O157:H7 IS HERE TO STAY

Since the initial 1982 outbreak of *E. coli* O157:H7, these infections have become one of the leading causes of diarrheal disease and food-borne outbreaks in the world. In addition, the *E. coli* O157:H7 bacterium is capable of contaminating water, other beverages, and various external environments, as is evidenced by the many outbreaks that have been reported to the CDC since 1990 (Table 1.1). In the United States alone, *E. coli* O157:H7 outbreaks occur regularly, affecting at least 20,000 people and killing 250 people per year.[10] This is clearly a public health problem that requires our attention.

2
What Is *E. coli*?

Once we understand the biology of Escherichia coli,
we will understand the biology of an elephant.

—Jacques Monod,
1965 winner of the Nobel Prize
for Physiology or Medicine

Escherichia coli (*E. coli*) is a type of **bacterium** (plural is *bacteria*)—a tiny singled-celled organism that can live in many different environments. Bacteria are found in the soil and water as well as on living organisms, including plants, people, and animals. Some bacteria can even survive in very strange places, such as hot springs, volcanoes, oceans, glaciers, and clouds. In some cases, bacteria are considered **pathogens**, or disease-causing organisms, because they can cause infections in people. However, they can also live on a human being without harming the person, in a relationship referred to as **commensalism**. In this situation, the bacteria obtain food and benefits from people without causing any kind of disease or damage. *E. coli* is often a commensal organism, but it also can cause a variety of diseases in humans.

AN IMPORTANT DISCOVERY

E. coli is a **prokaryote**, one of the smallest and most common groups of organisms in existence. Theodor Escherich, a German **bacteriologist**, or scientist who studies bacteria, first identified *E. coli* in 1885 in stool specimens collected from babies with enteritis.[1] *Enteritis* refers to an inflammation of the intestine that can cause stomach pain, nausea, vomiting, and diarrhea in people. At the time, this was a very significant

(continued on page 18)

BACTERIA'S FAMILY TREE

Cells are the basic unit of life. They contain all the important ingredients for an organism's survival and growth. All living organisms are divided into six separate kingdoms based on their physical appearance and structure: Eubacteria, Archaebacteria, Protista, Plantae, Fungae, and Animalia. Each kingdom is separated further by the cellular characteristics of the organisms within them. Most **unicellular** organisms are part of the Eubacteria (bacteria) and Archaebacteria kingdoms, whereas organisms from the Plantae (plants), Fungae (fungi), and Animalia (animals) kingdoms are **multicellular**, or composed of many cells. Bacteria are prokaryotes, whereas the unicellular Protists (Protista kingdom) and all other multicellular organisms are **eukaryotes**. The latter are more complex and are made up of multiple cells that need to work together (Figure 2.1). Each cell has a specific function involved in the organism's growth and survival. In contrast, unicellular organisms contain all the information that they need to live right inside one cell.[a]

After the electron microscope was invented in 1932, scientists could visually observe the differences between bacteria and multicellular organisms. Specifically, in prokaryotes, the genetic material that allows bacteria to survive is free-flowing throughout the **cytoplasm**, the gel-like liquid inside the cell.[b] In eukaryotes, the genetic material is contained inside a **nucleus**.

a. The University of Arizona. The Biology Project, 1999. Available online at *http://www.biology.arizona.edu/cell_bio/tutorials/pev/page1.html;* Ramel, G. Earth-Life Web Productions, 2003. Available online at *http://www.earthlife.net/cells.html.*

b. Stanier, R. Y., and C. B. van Niel. "The Main Outlines of Bacterial Classification." *Journal of Bacteriology* 42 (1941): 437–466.

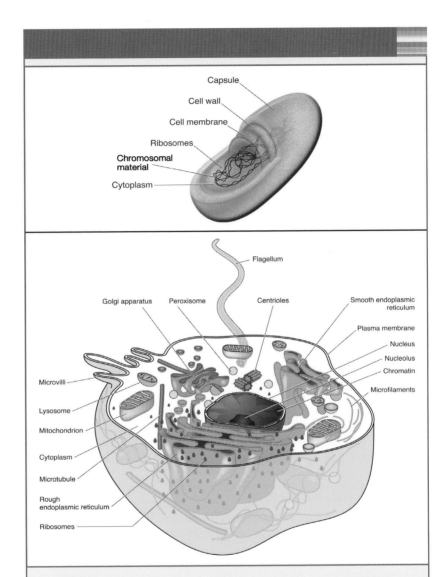

Capsule
Cell wall
Cell membrane
Ribosomes
Chromosomal material
Cytoplasm

Flagellum
Golgi apparatus   Peroxisome   Centrioles   Smooth endoplasmic reticulum
Plasma membrane
Nucleus
Nucleolus
Chromatin
Microvilli
Microfilaments
Lysosome
Mitochondrion
Cytoplasm
Microtubule
Rough endoplasmic reticulum
Ribosomes

Figure 2.1 A prokaryotic cell (top) contains chromosomal material (DNA) that is free-flowing throughout the cell and is not enclosed in a nucleus. Bacteria are prokaryotes. A typical eukaryotic cell (bottom) contains chromosomes (chromatin) within a nucleus that is separated from the cytoplasm. All animal and human cells are eukaryotes.

(continued from page 15)

finding because it identified *E. coli* as the cause of a specific disease. The bacterium was initially named *Bacterium coli*, but this was later changed to *Escherichia coli*, in honor of Escherich. Today, more is known about *E. coli* than about any other living organism, primarily because it has been studied the most.

THE *E. COLI* FAMILY

E. coli belongs to the *Escherichia* genus and is a well-known member of the Enterobacteriaceae family of bacteria. Enterobacteriaceae are commonly referred to as the enteric bacteria, or bacteria that can survive in the **gastrointestinal (GI) tract**, which consists of the digestive system structures (oral cavity, esophagus, stomach, intestines, rectum, and anus). Other members of the Enterobacteriaceae family include *Klebsiella*, *Shigella*, and *Salmonella*. The latter two are commonly associated with **food-borne diseases**, or diseases that are caused by organisms present in food or water. *Klebsiella* bacteria, on the other hand, can cause diseases ranging from urinary tract infections to pneumonia. *E. coli* is a straight **gram-negative** rod that can grow with (aerobically) or without (anaerobically) oxygen or air (Figure 2.2). The ability to grow in both conditions categorizes *E. coli* as a **facultative anaerobe**.

WHAT'S IN A CELL?

E. coli, like all bacterial cells, carries inside itself the information it needs for survival and growth. Each cell is small and composed of numerous structures. Inside the cell is a gel-like liquid material called the cytoplasm. The cytoplasm contains one circular **deoxyribonucleic acid (DNA)** molecule. DNA is a double-stranded molecule that encodes the genetic material that is unique to every organism.

In humans, DNA composition differences can cause one person to have brown hair and another person to have blond hair. Although bacteria have differences in their

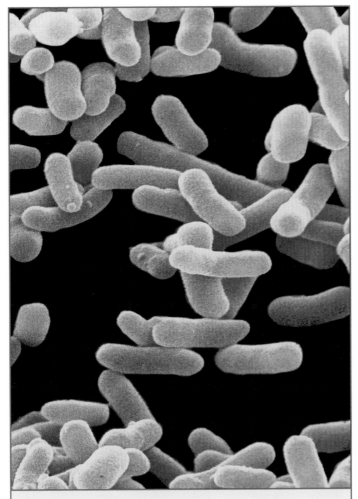

Figure 2.2 *Escherichia coli* are gram-negative rods, as can be seen in this electron micrograph.

DNA composition, too, these differences are often not noticeable. In bacterial cells, the DNA makes copies of itself in order to reproduce and create a new cell, referred to as a **daughter cell**. This technique is called **cell division**, and it can take place very rapidly under appropriate conditions. In fact, it is estimated that bacteria can divide once every 20 minutes.

(continued on page 22)

THE GRAM STAIN

Bacteria are divided into two groups based on their appearance after a Gram stain test has been performed. Christian Gram developed the Gram stain, a common laboratory technique used today, in 1884. Gram was a young physician from Denmark who noticed that certain bacteria turned violet after he stained them with methyl violet dye and an iodine solution, then washed them off with alcohol. He also saw that other bacteria could not be stained in this way. The Gram stain is performed only slightly differently today. Those bacteria that retain the violet stain are considered **gram-positive** bacteria, whereas those that lose the violet dye and turn red (due to the presence of a counterstain) are called **gram-negative** (Figure 2.3). The difference in staining is attributed to differences in the composition of the cell wall (Figure 2.4).[a] *E. coli* and all members of the Enterobacteriaceae family are gram-negative bacteria.

a. Smith, H. R., and T. Cheasty. "Diarrhoeal Diseases due to *Escherichia coli* and *Aeromonas*." *Topley and Wilson's Microbiology and Microbial Infections*, eds. L. Collier, A. Balows, and M. Sussman. London: Oxford University Press, 1998.

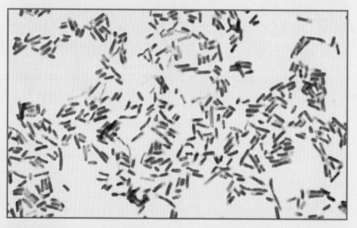

Figure 2.3 This photograph of *E. coli* (taken with a light microscope and magnified 400 times) shows the red color of the bacteria when stained using the Gram stain technique. *E. coli* appear red because they are gram-negative.

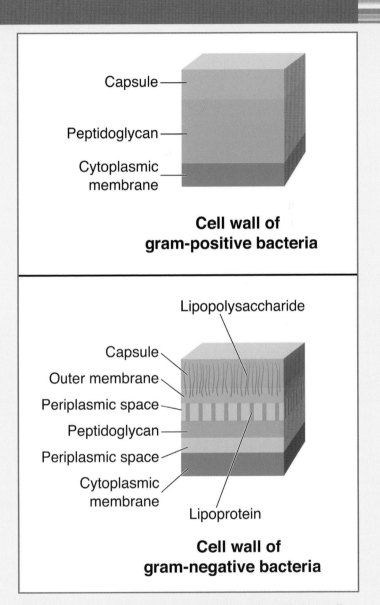

Capsule

Peptidoglycan

Cytoplasmic
membrane

**Cell wall of
gram-positive bacteria**

Lipopolysaccharide

Capsule

Outer membrane

Periplasmic space

Peptidoglycan

Periplasmic space

Cytoplasmic
membrane

Lipoprotein

**Cell wall of
gram-negative bacteria**

Figure 2.4 These diagrams show how the cell membrane, cell wall, and outer membrane of gram-negative and gram-positive bacteria differ. Bacteria react to the Gram stain differently depending on the composition of their outer layers.

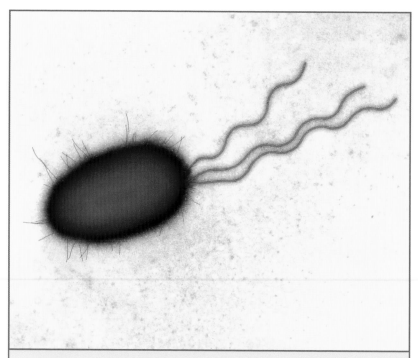

Figure 2.5 Shown here, at a magnification of x3,515, is an *Escherichia coli* bacterium with three tail-like flagella that it uses to propel itself through the environment.

(continued from page 19)

Daughter cells are initially identical to the original bacterial cell unless a genetic **mutation**—an alteration or change in the genetic material of a cell—takes place during division.

A thin **cell membrane** envelops the bacterial cell. Outside the cell membrane of bacteria, a very rigid **cell wall** acts as a protective barrier. While the rigidity causes the bacteria to be rather inflexible, it also makes the cell stronger and provides protection from harmful environments. The cell wall consists of two structures: a fluid-filled area called the periplasmic gel that contains a layer of peptidoglycan, and an **outer membrane** (refer again to Figure 2.4 on page 21). The outer membrane is composed of proteins and fatty acid substances called **phospholipids** and **lipopolysaccharides**. Lipopolysaccharides extend out of the bacterial cell wall and act as **endotoxins**, which are responsible for many of the damaging effects of gram-negative bacteria. The outer membrane components work together to enhance the bacterium's survival and facilitate the development of disease.

In addition to the outer membrane components, many *E. coli* also have **flagella**, or tail-like appendages that extend from the membrane (Figure 2.5). Flagella can propel the bacterium to suitable environments, and are important for bacterial survival.

3

A Plethora of Diseases

For the most part, diseases are grouped into two distinct categories: infectious or chronic. An **infectious disease** is caused by a micro-organism, such as a bacterium, **virus, parasite**, or **fungus**, whereas **chronic diseases** are conditions that can last for an extended period of time and are generally noninfectious in origin. Some chronic diseases, however, are actually triggered by a pathogen, or infectious agent (Table 3.1).

CHARACTERISTICS OF INFECTIOUS DISEASES

In 1998, infectious diseases were ranked second, following heart disease (cardiovascular disease), as the leading cause of death worldwide (Figure 3.1). At that time, infectious diseases caused approximately 25% of all deaths in the world, which translates to about 17.3 million deaths per year.[1] This number appears to be increasing; infectious diseases accounted for 36% of all deaths in 2002, and according to the World Health Organization, infectious disease deaths in Africa outnumbered noninfectious disease deaths.[2]

In contrast to infectious diseases, chronic diseases represent conditions that last for an extended period of time and are not caused by a specific pathogen. Cancer is a well-known example of a chronic disease. It is caused by numerous factors that work together in a complex and unknown way. In general, certain cells inside a person with cancer have been reprogrammed to develop into a tumor, or abnormal mass of cells. These cells lose their ability to function in a normal manner, and can spread to other parts of the body. If the spread is not controlled, it can lead to death. Other common chronic diseases include leukemia, multiple sclerosis (MS), and Parkinson's disease.

Table 3.1 Examples of common diseases separated by disease category. Some chronic diseases can develop following an infection with certain pathogens

Common disease	Disease symptoms/ characteristics	Disease Category		Pathogen
		Infectious	Chronic	
Bloody diarrhea	Bloody stools and diarrhea, chills, dehydration, and stomach cramps. Can cause death in certain people (e.g., infants and the elderly).	X		Bacteria (e.g., *E. coli* O157:H7), viruses (e.g., enterovirus) parasites (e.g., *Giardia lamblia*)
Hemolytic uremic syndrome (HUS)	Diarrhea-associated symptoms followed by more severe disease (e.g., kidney failure) that can lead to death.	X	X	Bacteria (e.g., *E. coli* O157:H7)
Acquired immunodeficiency syndrome (AIDS)	Weakened immune response, prone to infection, weakness, fatigue, arthritis, dementia and other neurological complications that lead to death.	X	X	Virus (human immunodeficiency virus (HIV))
Lung cancer	Decreased lung capacity and breathing difficulties that can lead to death.		X	None identified so far
Parkinson's disease	Altered mental status, speech and movement difficulties, tremors, and swallowing difficulties that can lead to death.		X	None identified so far
Hepatocellular carcinoma	Liver cancer that contributes to poor liver function and eventual death.	X	X	Viruses (e.g., hepatitis B virus [HBV])
Meningitis	Blood infection that causes swelling in the membranes surrounding the brain and spinal cord. Symptoms include fever, chills, headache, altered mental status and delirium, and can lead to coma and/or death.	X		Bacteria (e.g., *E. coli*, *Neisseria meningitidis*) viruses (e.g., West Nile virus)

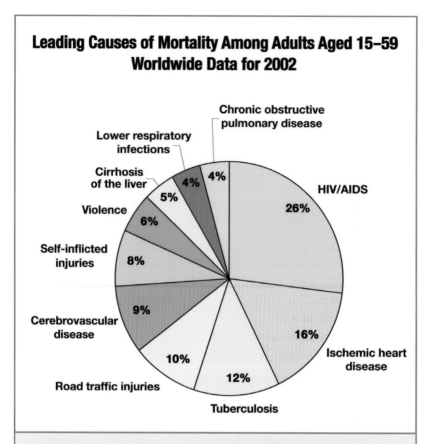

**Leading Causes of Mortality Among Adults Aged 15–59
Worldwide Data for 2002**

Chronic obstructive pulmonary disease

Lower respiratory infections

Cirrhosis of the liver

Violence

Self-inflicted injuries

Cerebrovascular disease

Road traffic injuries

HIV/AIDS 26%

Ischemic heart disease 16%

Tuberculosis 12%

4% 4%

5%

6%

8%

9%

10%

Figure 3.1 According to 2002 data from the World Health Organization, several infectious diseases were included in the top ten leading causes of death list. HIV/AIDS and tuberculosis ranked first and third among 15- to 59-year-olds, respectively, while respiratory infections ranked fourth among the elderly.

Interestingly, the origin of some chronic diseases is a pathogen, such as a virus or bacterium. Human papillomavirus (HPV) infection, for example, can lead to the development of cervical cancer, wheras *E. coli* O157:H7 infection can cause severe kidney disease. Similarly, infection with the hepatitis C virus (HCV) can contribute to liver damage and eventually cause cancer of the liver (or hepatocellular carcinoma) in some

(continued on page 30)

THE CONTINUOUS THREAT OF EMERGING INFECTIOUS DISEASES

Emerging infectious diseases, defined as newly identified or re-emerging diseases, are cause for great concern in today's society. When a previously unrecognized pathogen comes in contact with a susceptible population, there is serious potential for devastating consequences. The outbreak of severe acute respiratory syndrome (SARS), first discovered in China in the late part of 2002, provides a current example. SARS took China by surprise. More than 7,000 people got sick and over 800 died within less than a year. SARS also spread rapidly to other nations by infected travelers. The United States, for example, reported 211 SARS cases as of July 2003, while Canada reported 251 cases and 41 deaths.[a] Numerous public health measures were taken to prevent further transmission of SARS. For example, in China, stores closed, employees stayed home from work, children stayed home from school, and public transportation systems shut down. All of these measures obviously had an enormous economic impact. Scientists now believe that the pathogen responsible for SARS is a previously unknown type of coronavirus. Other types of coronaviruses include some that cause the common cold.

E. coli O157:H7–associated disease is also considered an emerging infection, since this type of E. coli was not observed in humans until 1982. This newly discovered type of E. coli is now a major cause of diarrheal disease outbreaks worldwide. Some suggest that the emergence of E. coli O157:H7 as a human pathogen occurred because the bacterium changed or evolved in a way that made it more pathogenic, thereby increasing its ability to cause disease.[b] Many different factors that contribute to the development of emerging infectious diseases have been identified. Some examples are highlighted in Table 3.2.

a. United States Department of Health and Human Services, Centers for Disease Control and Prevention, Office of Communication, Division of Media Relations. 2003. Available online at http://www.cdc.gov/od/oc/media/pressrel/r030717a.htm.

b. Whittam, T. S., E. A. McGraw, and S. D. Reid. "Pathogenic Escherichia coli O157:H7: A model for Emerging Infectious Diseases." Emerging Infections: Biomedical Research Reports, ed. R. M. Krause. New York: Academic Press, 1998.

Table 3.2 Factors associated with the development of emerging infectious diseases

Factor associated with emerging infections	Disease example	Pathogen	Geographic location	Reason for emergence
First contact with susceptible humans	AIDS	Human immuno-deficiency virus (HIV)	Central Africa	The development of a large highway connected numerous towns and enabled previously separated people to interact with each other.
Mixing of human populations	SARS	Coronavirus	Toronto, Canada	Tourists infected with the virus returned from China and spread the infection locally.
Poor water quality	Severe diarrhea	*Cryptosporidium parvum*	Wisconsin	Sewage-contaminated drinking water was distributed to city residents.
Bad weather	Malaria	Malaria-infected mosquito	Africa	Global warming that causes temperature increases provides a perfect environment for disease-carrying mosquitoes.
Human activities that set the stage for disease	Plague	*Yersinia pestis* bacterium	Surat, India	An overabundance of emergency aid (e.g., food) delivered to India following an earthquake and flood caused an infestation of disease-carrying rats.

Factor associated with emerging infections	Disease example	Pathogen	Geographic location	Reason for emergence
Urbanization and/or deforestation	Dengue hemorrhagic fever	Dengue-infected mosquito	Asia	Pools of water left over at construction sites make ideal breeding grounds for disease-carrying mosquitoes.
Unstable political conditions/breakdown in the public health system	Tuberculosis	*Mycobacterium tuberculosis* bacterium	Russia	A disruption in the government's social structure (e.g., during war) takes key resources away from combating infectious diseases.
Human beliefs	Whooping cough	*Bordetella pertussis* bacterium	Michigan	Public health officials find it difficult to vaccinate children and members of specific communities that do not believe in the vaccination (e.g., the Amish).
Contaminated food supply	Bloody diarrhea	*E. coli* O157:H7 bacterium	Washington	Contaminated ground beef that was not cooked properly.
Changes in the microorganism	The "flu"	*Influenzavirus*	Worldwide	Changes in the genetic makeup of the influenza virus make it more adaptable to humans who had previous exposure to other influenza virus types.
Living conditions	Sexually transmitted disease	Bacteria (e.g., *Neisseria gonorrheae*) viruses (e.g., HIV)	Mumbai, India	Poverty prevents infected people from getting appropriate treatments; thus, they can transmit various infections to others via sexual activity.

(*continued from page 26*)

people. Clearly, in these situations, the long-term complications associated with the infection are much more debilitating and severe than the primary infection.

HOW ARE INFECTIOUS DISEASES TRANSMITTED?

Infectious diseases can be transmitted between people by many different pathways. One common pathway is **aerosol transmission**, which occurs when an infected person sneezes or coughs, expelling infectious microorganisms into the air. "The flu," an infection caused by *influenzaviruses*, is an example of a common infectious disease spread in this manner. Microorganisms transmitted via the air tend to be highly contagious and can infect a large number of people in a short amount of time.

Disease-causing microorganisms also can be transmitted by direct, person-to-person transmission, which includes sexual contact. This pathway relies on the microorganism's ability to survive in body fluids such as blood. The human immunodeficiency virus (HIV) that causes acquired immunodeficiency syndrome (AIDS) is primarily transmitted by sexual activity. It also can be spread by drug users who share contaminated needles. Before blood-screening procedures were established, some people acquired HIV through blood transfusions, and, in rare cases, health-care workers acquired HIV when they were injured with contaminated syringes.

Contamination of the food or water supply also can lead to the transmission of infectious diseases. *E. coli* O157:H7 infections can occur when people ingest food or water contaminated with the bacterium, whereas cholera—another acute diarrheal illness—results when people drink water contaminated with the *Vibrio cholerae* bacterium. In 1993, the parasite *Cryptosporidium parvum* caused a major diarrheal disease outbreak in Milwaukee, Wisconsin, after it contaminated the public water supply.

These food- and water-borne pathogens are transmitted to people by the **fecal-oral route**. That is, they enter the body through the mouth and take up residence in the gastrointes-tinal tract. The pathogens can then be eliminated in feces, primarily as diarrhea, and can survive elsewhere in the environment (e.g., in water). People who come in contact with contaminated environments or animals (such as cows) are more likely to become infected. This is particularly true for children, who do not routinely wash their hands and, therefore, can easily spread the bacteria from their hands to their mouths and, from there, to the gastrointestinal tract.

Lastly, indirect transmission via a **vector**, or an organism that transmits a disease, also occurs regularly. Lyme disease—a disorder that causes flu-like symptoms, a rash, neurological complications, and arthritis in some people—results when a specific type of tick carrying the *Borrelia burgdorferi* bacterium bites and infects a person. Mosquitoes are the culprit in many other well-known vector-borne infections, including malaria, West Nile virus, and dengue hemorrhagic fever.

THE TRANSMISSION CYCLE

Transmission from one animal, human, or environment to another depends on several interconnected components. The transmission cycle for an *E. coli* O157:H7 infection begins with a pathogen that has the ability to cause disease in humans. The pathogen originates from a reservoir—a specific environment (such as water) or organism (such as a cow) that provides nutrients that allow the pathogen to grow and survive. Next, a pathogen must come in contact with a susceptible person via one of the many different transmission modes (such as the fecal-oral route). Most pathogens require a specific entry site into a person, such as the mouth or blood, to enhance survival. Transmission to others occurs when a person develops symptoms that reintroduce the pathogen back into the environment or reservoir (such as a diarrheal episode in a swimming pool), thereby allowing it to come in contact with other susceptible people.

WHAT ARE THE MOST COMMON INFECTIOUS DISEASES?

Evidence suggests that infectious diseases have been affecting human populations since before 430 B.C.[3] Today, our society continues to battle infectious diseases, though the types of infections have changed over time. For example, the plague caused by the *Yersinia pestis* bacterium caused the death of up to 24 million people during the 14th century.[4] Smallpox, caused by the variola virus, and syphilis, caused by the *Treponema pallidum* bacterium, also are considered historical pathogens, since they were first detected in the 14th and 15th centuries, respectively. These days, the plague occurs only rarely, smallpox has been completely eliminated from human populations, and, although syphilis remains a problem in some areas, it is not nearly as common as it once was. Other equally severe infectious diseases, such as diarrheal diseases and influenza, however, have emerged over time to take the place of these illnesses. A new distribution of infectious diseases has resulted, making it clear that infectious diseases are here to stay (Figure 3.2).

DIARRHEA: A COMMON INFECTIOUS DISEASE

Diarrheal disease, a major public health concern worldwide, is characterized by the production of frequent liquid stools. A diagnosis is generally made if an individual passes three or more liquid stools in a 24-hour period.[5]

Today, **diarrhea** is considered one of the top causes of death in children under the age of five. In 1996, it was estimated that diarrhea was causing approximately 1.9 million deaths per year worldwide.[6] Recent estimates reveal that diarrheal diseases ranked second out of the top 10 leading causes of childhood deaths worldwide.[7] Waterborne infections that contribute to diarrheal disease cause up to 80% of all infectious diseases worldwide and 90% of infections in developing countries.[8]

Starting in the early 1980s, great efforts were made to decrease the number of deaths from diarrheal disease. Diarrhea-associated

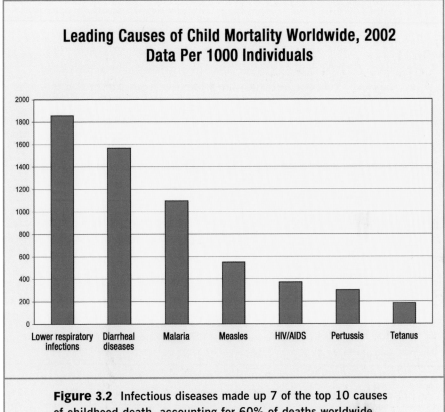

Leading Causes of Child Mortality Worldwide, 2002
Data Per 1000 Individuals

Figure 3.2 Infectious diseases made up 7 of the top 10 causes of childhood death, accounting for 60% of deaths worldwide. Diarrheal diseases caused death in 1,566,000 children around the world in 2002, and ranked second behind lower respiratory infections as the leading cause of childhood death.

deaths are primarily caused by the severe dehydration that follows prolonged diarrhea. Prevention practices aimed at rehydrating patients have resulted in lower rates of disease in both developing and developed countries.[9] Today, those who die from diarrheal diseases are generally very young or very old, have a more severe form of persistent or bloody diarrhea called dysentery,[10] and live in developing countries.

Diarrhea is also a very common short-term illness in both children and adults. In developing countries, some young children can have up to 10 episodes of diarrhea per year, although the frequency in developed countries is lower.[11] Several settings in developed countries, however, are more likely to have higher rates of diarrheal disease. These include day-care centers, hospitals, and nursing homes, which are affected more frequently because person-to-person transmission risks are high and the very young and the very old are more susceptible to infections.[12]

THE ROLE OF POVERTY

The high rate of diarrheal disease in developing nations can likely be attributed to the high number of people living in poverty. Recent estimates suggest that approximately 1.5 billion people worldwide live in poverty and make less than $1.00 a day; this number is increasing, particularly in developing countries,[13] such as some countries in Latin America and Africa. Poverty has a tremendous impact on all infectious diseases, because those measures that help halt the spread of disease, including appropriate sanitary conditions, housing, proper maintenance of public water systems and latrines, disease treatment, and important prevention practices (e.g., mosquito repellant), are all costly.

Poverty occurs in developed countries, too. In the United States, for instance, nearly 13% of Americans live below the poverty line. Those Americans most vulnerable to the scourge of infectious diseases are the homeless, who are thought to comprise approximately 1 million people.

WHAT CAUSES DIARRHEA?

Because many different microorganisms, including various bacteria, viruses, and parasites, can cause diarrhea, it is extremely difficult to study the disease itself. Therefore, investigators classify diarrheal disease by the causative agent. Enterotoxigenic *E. coli* (ETEC) bacteria have been implicated as the cause of most diarrheal episodes in approximately 13 different developing countries, followed by *Giardia lamblia*, a parasite; *Campylobacter* bacteria; a virus called rotavirus; the *Cryptosporidium parvum* parasite; and various *Shigella* bacteria.[14]

E. COLI TYPES THAT CAUSE SEVERE DIARRHEA

E. coli types can cause disease in people by different mechanisms and can contribute to a wide range of symptoms. Researchers found the first case of *E. coli*–associated disease in the early 1920s; it was thought to cause diarrhea in infants.[15] Since this discovery, five specific *E. coli* types have been discovered, all of which contribute to severe diarrheal disease. Other types may exist that have yet to be identified.

A complicated naming system was developed to distinguish each type of diarrhea-associated *E. coli*. In most cases, the name reflects the type of disease that *E. coli* causes or the mechanism by which it causes disease. For example, *E. coli* O157:H7 is also referred to as **enterohemorrhagic *E. coli***, or EHEC, because it commonly causes bloody diarrhea. *Entero* comes from the Greek word *enteron*, meaning "intestine," while *hemorrhagic* means "bleeding." Therefore, EHEC is defined as *E. coli* bacteria that cause intestinal bleeding. The other *E. coli* types include enteropathogenic *E. coli* (EPEC), enteroadherent *E. coli* (EAEC), enteroinvasive *E. coli* (EIEC), and enterotoxigenic *E. coli* (ETEC).

In order to classify the circulating *E. coli* types further, a novel typing method was developed in 1944 that assesses the type of *E. coli* **polysaccharide** present on the outer surface of the cell (capsule). This is referred to as the **serotype**.[16] Approximately 173 *E. coli* serotypes exist, ranging from O1 to O173.[17] *E. coli* O157:H7, for example, represents the 157th serotype. The use of serotyping to distinguish between diarrhea-associated *E. coli* types helps determine whether particular strains are part of an outbreak. Other type-specific characteristics also have been identified and will be discussed in later chapters.

EHEC-ASSOCIATED INFECTIONS

EHEC, which includes the infamous *E. coli* O157:H7, is known to cause diarrhea; hemorrhagic colitis, or grossly bloody diarrhea preceded by a fever and stomach cramps; and hemolytic uremic syndrome (HUS), a serious long-term complication that primarily affects children. HUS causes abnormal bleeding, kidney failure, and nervous system problems. Adults and children also may develop thrombotic thrombocytopenic purpura (TTP), a severe and often fatal condition similar to HUS.

EHEC are different from other diarrhea-associated *E. coli* types in that they possess a potent toxin called the **Shiga toxin**. In some reports, Shiga toxin–producing *E. coli* (STEC) are also called Vero cytotoxin–producing *E. coli* (VTEC). Researchers have determined that the Shiga toxins released by *E. coli* O157:H7 damage the vascular endothelial cells—the cells of the tissues that line the internal organs—thereby facilitating severe disease.

ETEC-ASSOCIATED INFECTIONS

ETEC strains are a very common cause of diarrhea worldwide and are often associated with **gastroenteritis**—an inflammation of the stomach and intestinal lining that causes nausea, diarrhea, stomach pain, and weakness. Gastroenteritis in travelers, called traveler's diarrhea (also referred to as Montezuma's revenge, the GI trots, and Turista), is caused by bacteria in the local water or food. The *E. coli* that contaminates food is generally different from the *E. coli* that a person contacts regularly at home and is often present at much higher frequencies. This contact with a new *E. coli* type, combined with the physical stresses associated with traveling, may cause a person to become very sick. In addition to diarrhea and loose stools, traveler's diarrhea is associated with stomach cramps, bloating, gas, nausea, fever, weakness, and dehydration that lasts between three and seven days.[18] Although people who suffer from this condition often feel miserable, traveler's diarrhea is rarely life-threatening.

ETEC also are associated with severe diarrhea in children of developing nations who have just been weaned from breastfeeding. In this situation, ETEC usually affects between 10 and 30% of infants. The transmission of ETEC to these children occurs primarily through the food and water in areas with endemic infections and high rates of ETEC-associated disease.

NON-DIARRHEAL INFECTIONS CAUSED BY *E. COLI*

In addition to diarrheal disease, *E. coli* also causes a number of other diseases, including urinary tract infections (UTIs). A UTI results from an infection of the bladder or other structures within the urinary tract. UTIs can develop in both men and women, although they are more common in women. The *E. coli* that cause UTIs are referred to as **uropathogenic *E. coli* (UPEC)**. Several studies have demonstrated that UPEC are very different from the diarrhea-associated *E. coli* strains. In some people, infection with UPEC can lead to pyelonephritis, a serious inflammation of the kidneys. Even though pyelonephritis is not as common as UTI, it is much more severe and can lead to death, particularly in children.

E. coli also can cause infections outside the gastrointestinal tract. Respiratory infections such as pneumonia can develop, but these are considered **opportunistic infections**—infections caused by a microorganism that does not normally cause disease. In general, most people can fight *E. coli* infections with their natural immune system defenses; however, some people, particularly children, those with existing medical conditions, and the elderly, often have a weaker immune response. Therefore, these individuals have more difficulty combating the infection and are more susceptible to long-term complications.

Newborn babies are extremely vulnerable to all infectious agents, primarily because of their underdeveloped immune system. When infected with *E. coli*, newborns can sometimes develop bacterial meningitis. Meningitis is a serious condition characterized by inflammation of the meninges, or the membranes that surround the brain and spinal cord. This condition can be fatal and can leave survivors with long-term disabilities, including deafness, blindness, and brain damage.

WHERE DOES *E. COLI* RESIDE?

E. coli has very specific preferences regarding the environment in which it lives. It is most attracted to the human tissues that line the gastrointestinal tract. These tissues are also referred to as mucous membranes. In a phase called **colonization**, *E. coli* bacteria use specific characteristics and structural components to attach to these membranes. Most people are colonized with *E. coli* bacteria and do not show any signs of infection. In other words, they have **asymptomatic colonization**. Initially, *E. coli* was perceived to be a pathogen that caused diarrheal disease in infants; however, this perception was altered after researchers identified *E. coli* in the stool of healthy babies and adults.[19] Today, it is understood that *E. coli* and millions of other microorganisms live in the human body and are considered to be part of the **normal flora**— microorganisms residing in the human body that produce essential molecules and protect the body from invasion by disease-causing pathogens.

Because *E. coli* prefer to live in the tissues of the gastrointestinal tract, it is not surprising that the diseases caused by the bacterium tend to affect this area. Some common complications that result from an *E. coli* infection include diarrhea and stomach pain, though these may differ in each person.

E. coli also can spread to the **genitourinary tract**, which consists of the kidneys, ureters, bladder, urethra, and reproductive organs like the vagina. In more deadly situations, *E. coli* can enter the bloodstream and be distributed to other vulnerable organs, including the brain, heart, and lungs.

HOW IMPORTANT IS ASYMPTOMATIC COLONIZATION?

Although the *E. coli* and other bacteria that make up a person's normal flora are thought to be different from disease-causing strains, this is not always true. A well-known example of this involved an outbreak of typhoid fever in New York City in the early 1900s. Typhoid fever is a very serious condition that can cause fever, weakness, headache, chills, delirium, stomach cramping, diarrhea, constipation, and cough, and can contribute to many long-term complications, including bone and muscle damage and heart failure. It is caused by the *Salmonella typhi* bacterium and is transmitted to people through food or the fecal-oral route. Eventually, health-care officials traced the original outbreak, consisting of 53 cases, to a woman named Mary Mallon, who became known as "Typhoid Mary."

Mallon was a healthy Irish cook who visited many homes in the city to cook meals for the residents. In order to determine whether she was the source of the outbreak, her stool was cultured for the presence of the bacteria. Although she showed no signs of infection herself, her stool was positive for *S. typhi*. As a result, she was prohibited from working in the food service industry for three years, until 1910. After this, Mallon disappeared from the city and changed her identity. Approximately two years later, health officials traced another typhoid fever outbreak consisting of 200 cases in New York and New Jersey to her. Mallon was again found to be asymptomatically colonized with *S. typhi* and was probably excreting the bacteria in her feces regularly. Since handwashing was not as commonplace in the early 1900s as it is today, Mallon was likely contaminating the food after she had a bowel movement.

Source: Soper, G. A. "The Curious Case of Typhoid Mary." *Academic Medicine: Journal of the Association of American Medical Colleges* 15 (1939): 698–712.

4

Epidemiology of *E. coli* Infections

Understanding the frequency and distribution of each disease type throughout the world is an important first step in eradicating infectious diseases. In 1801, Edward Jenner was the first to suggest that infectious diseases could actually be eradicated. At that time, he spoke of "the annihilation of the Small Pox." This implied that humans had the power to eliminate this deadly viral disease, as well as other infectious diseases, permanently from the face of the Earth. No one knew, however, just how difficult this task would be. After millions of dollars were spent and millions of people were immunized with the smallpox **vaccine**, the disease was finally eradicated from human populations 176 years later.

Disease eradication is often very difficult to achieve for numerous reasons. One example is that changes in the pathogen and/or changes in the pathogen's location relative to human populations can stifle control efforts. Despite this, eradication remains an important goal of health-care organizations worldwide. To date, smallpox eradication has been the only completely successful program, in that the disease no longer exists outside of laboratories. Numerous other eradication programs, including those targeting the parasitic diseases hookworm and malaria, have failed; however, the frequency of these diseases has declined following intense eradication efforts (Table 4.1).

Failed eradication programs have illustrated to scientists that it is essential to understand fully how the targeted disease affects humans and in what capacity. For example, gaining a better understanding of the causative agent, its transmission dynamics and life cycle,

Table 4.1: Examples of unsuccessful eradication programs targeting specific infectious diseases. To date, smallpox remains the only infectious disease to be successfully eliminated from human populations

Disease	Infectious agent	Clinical illness	Type and date of eradication program	Country/region of interest	Some reasons for failure	Consequences
Poliomyelitis[1]	Poliovirus	Minor symptoms in 90% of cases; paralysis and meningitis occur in < 3% of cases.	Vaccination (1996–2002)	Nigeria	Rumors about the safety of the polio vaccine forced health-care workers to suspend vaccination programs.	Reintroduction of poliovirus into previously unaffected areas, which caused an increase in the number of cases.
Yaws[2]	Treponema pallidum bacterium	Contagious skin lesions; can cause crippling and disfigurement; primarily affects children.	Mass antibiotic (penicillin) treatment of affected individuals (1950s and 1960s)	Tropical areas (e.g., in parts of Africa, Asia, and Latin America)	People with latent, or not yet symptomatic, infections got ill after mass treatment of their community. Some members were asymptomatic and received no treatment.	The infection continued to spread in the community despite the mass treatment.
Measles[3]	Measles virus	Highly contagious producing a distinct rash, fever, cough; more severe in infants and adults.	Mass vaccination of 9-month-olds to 14-year-olds (1987–1997)	São Paulo, Brazil	Not all children were vaccinated, cases were imported from affected areas, and high population density promoted spread.	The many susceptible children enhanced the spread of disease, quickly resulting in over 20,000 cases.
Malaria[2]	Parasites (Plasmodium sp) carried and transmitted by mosquitoes	High fever that can lead to shock, organ failure, and death; fatality rates exceed 10% in some areas.	WHO Global Malaria Eradication Campaign spent $1.4 billion to increase insecticide use and distribute anti-malaria medications (1955–1965)	Tropical areas in Africa	The campaign was costly and time-consuming, mosquitoes developed resistance to insecticides, and parasites developed resistance to medications.	The campaign was revised to focus on malaria control versus eradication in 1969 after billions were spent and disease persisted.

[1] Centers for Disease Control and Prevention. "Progress toward poliomyelitis eradication—Nigeria,January 2003–March 2004." *Morbidity and Mortality Weekly Report* 53, no.16 (2004): 343–346. Available online at *http://www.cdc.gov.*

[2] Centers for Disease Control and Prevention. "Recommendations and Reports." *Morbidity and Mortality Weekly Report* 43, no. RR16 (1993): 1–25. Available online at *http://www.cdc.gov.*

[3] Pan American Health Organization. "Update: São Paulo measles outbreak." *EPI newsletter* 20 (1998): 5–6.

and its mechanism of survival in humans is necessary to assess whether eradication efforts are feasible. Additionally, it is imperative to understand the distribution of the disease on a global scale. All of these topics fall under the science of **epidemiology**—the study of the occurrence, distribution, transmission, and prevention of disease in specific populations. Epidemiologists, individuals who study epidemiology, play a key role in enhancing our understanding of the disease

HISTORY OF EPIDEMIOLOGY

The Greek physician Hippocrates, considered the founder of human medicine, suggested in the 5th century B.C. that human disease is the result not only of one's internal environment, but also of one's external environment.[a] This observation suggests that numerous factors work together to cause human disease. These factors, often referred to as **risk factors**, may be related to the environment, the affected person (**host**), or the causative agent (pathogen). Examples of environmental factors include climate, land design, and sanitation practices, while factors specific to the host may include age, gender, nutritional status, and the type of immune response elicited. Factors specific to the pathogen may include particular components produced by the agent, such as the Shiga toxin produced by *E. coli* O157:H7, which facilitates disease development.[b]

In 1662, a British merchant named John Graunt made the first attempt to quantify disease patterns in a population. By researching the birth and death rates of people living in London, Graunt collected data that specifically provided information about human diseases.[c] This is the basis of epidemiology.[d]

Perhaps the most famous historical epidemiologist was a British physician named John Snow. In 1854, Snow wanted to determine why cholera, a deadly bacterial disease that causes severe diarrhea, was killing so many people in some London neighborhoods but not others. Although scientists had not yet process and identifying people who may be more susceptible to developing certain infections.

A common way that epidemiologists assess the distribution of specific diseases in a population and are alerted to the arrival of an emerging pathogen is by developing a **surveillance system**. These systems rely on the interactions of numerous people and institutions (e.g., health-care providers, clinical laboratories, public health officials, hospitals, and the public),

discovered the actual bacterium, *Vibrio cholerae*, at this time, Snow used standard epidemiological tools to determine the cause of the outbreak.

First, Snow visited the house of each family that had reported a cholera death during a certain time period. In an attempt to identify something that each family had in common, he interviewed all family members, and afterward, he plotted the distribution of the cholera-associated deaths (Figure 4.1).

Snow's findings revealed that the death rate from cholera was particularly high among people who got their water from a pump connected to a section of the Thames River that was contaminated with sewage. In contrast, people who used pumps that came from a cleaner portion of the river were free of the disease. After describing the frequency and distribution of cholera in London, Snow tested his hypothesis that cholera was being transmitted to people via a contaminated water pump by removing the handle from the suspected pump. The cholera outbreak ended immediately.

From this point on, epidemiology was referred to as the study of infectious disease **epidemics** caused by microorganisms or other infectious agents. Because non-infectious diseases, also known as chronic diseases, have increased in frequency over time, epidemiologists now study the distribution and causes of these types of diseases as

HISTORY OF EPIDEMIOLOGY *(continued)*

well. Today, the epidemiological methods used by Snow are essential in many fields outside epidemiology, including environmental studies and clinical medicine.

a. Hippocrates. "On Airs, Waters, and Places." *Medical Classics,* vol. 3, 1938.

b. The toxin produced by *E. coli* is formally called Shiga-like toxin because it resembles the toxin produced by *Shigella*, which is a closely related enteric pathogen. The toxin is often called Shiga toxin for simplicity.

c. Graunt, J. *Natural and Political Observations Made upon the Bills of Mortality: London, 1662.* Baltimore: Johns Hopkins University Press, 1939.

d. Hennekens, C. H., and J. E. Buring,. *Epidemiology in Medicine.* Boston/Toronto: Little Brown, 1987.

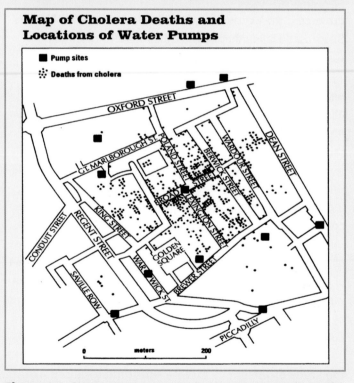

Map of Cholera Deaths and Locations of Water Pumps

■ Pump sites

∴ Deaths from cholera

Figure 4.1 Shown here is an example of a map created by John Snow. Each cholera-associated death in this section of London is represented as a dot. Based on the distribution of deaths, Snow was able to determine that a specific water pump was the source of the cholera outbreak.

located in distinct geographic areas, to survey and report disease information back to the epidemiologists. Data generated from surveillance systems allow epidemiologists to measure disease frequencies, monitor trends, make comparisons between geographic locations, and identify people and areas that are more prone to the development of the disease.

WHERE AND WHEN DO *E. COLI*–ASSOCIATED DIARRHEAL DISEASES OCCUR?

The frequency and distribution of *E. coli* infections vary by location and type of *E. coli* present in an environment. As with many other infectious diseases, *E. coli*–associated diarrheal disease occurs in developed countries like the United States, but is more common in developing countries where proper sanitation and hygiene practices, a clean water supply, basic education, and a well-funded public health system are often lacking.[2] In contrast, outbreaks of food-borne diarrheal disease associated with EHEC infections (e.g., *E. coli* O157:H7) are more common in the United States and other developed countries, with some exceptions (Figure 4.2). In the United States, *E. coli*–associated diseases also occur during the warmer months when the likelihood of food contamination is higher (e.g., at picnics; Figure 4.3).

EHEC INFECTIONS

EHEC-associated diseases are characterized by infection with Shiga toxin–producing *E. coli* (STEC). These strains, composed of serotypes O157:H7 and at least 20 non-O157:H7 strains, have become a major public health concern. The reported frequency, however, is not an accurate representation of the true frequency of EHEC, since many laboratories do not actively screen for the presence of the bacterium (Figure 4.4).

As discussed earlier, EHEC are mainly transmitted to people through contaminated food or water, and outbreaks often result. Infection with *E. coli* 0157:H7 is quite serious and leads to hospitalization in up to 40% of cases (Figure 4.5). Following episodes of severe, bloody diarrhea, some individuals will develop long-term complications, such as HUS, which causes death in 2% of those affected.[3] The majority of HUS cases occur in South America, particularly Argentina, where it is **endemic**. The incidence for various regions in the United States, Scotland, and Canada is estimated to be 8 cases per 100,000 people per year.[4] In the United States, 24 states

MEASURING DISEASE FREQUENCIES

The most basic measure of disease frequency is a count of the number of affected people. It is also important to know the size of the population at risk, or that could potentially be affected, and identify a specific period of time to be evaluated. The **prevalence**, calculated as the number of infected people divided by the total number of people in a given population, provides a very important measure. To determine whether a specific disease is increasing in frequency in a particular area, epidemiologists must be aware of the endemic disease level—the level of disease that is usually present in a given population. If the number of disease cases increases rapidly and significantly above the endemic level, then the situation is referred to as an epidemic or outbreak. A specific outbreak that occurs in multiple countries at the same time is called a **pandemic**. AIDS and SARS are examples of pandemics.

Another important measure of disease frequency is the **incidence**, or number of new infections in a given population during a specific time period. This differs from the prevalence in that it measures only new cases in an area and does not account for people who have had a given disease for a long period of time. For the most part, the incidence and prevalence vary by geographic location, population type and size, and pathogen.

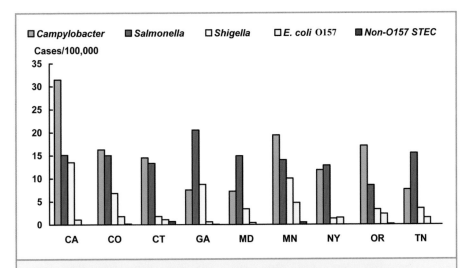

Figure 4.2 This graph shows the number (y-axis) of food-borne disease cases per 100,000 people in 2001. The letters on the x-axis represent the various states in the United States that are taking part in the CDC food-borne disease surveillance system. Shiga-like toxin producing *E. coli* are represented by the light blue and dark purple bars.

reported 249 cases of HUS in 2000; most cases were in young children (56% of whom were female) between June and September. The number of HUS cases has increased significantly since 1998, when only 17 states reported a total of 119 cases. Health officials attribute the increased number of cases to better surveillance methods rather than a real increase in disease frequency; however, underreporting is still an issue.[5]

EPEC INFECTIONS

In the 1940s, diarrheal disease outbreaks were very common in nurseries and hospitals during the winter months. These outbreaks were often severe and caused numerous deaths. An investigation in a London hospital identified the causative agent as *E. coli* O111,[6] while other investigations in Scotland found two strains—*E. coli* O111 and O55—to be at fault.[7] The

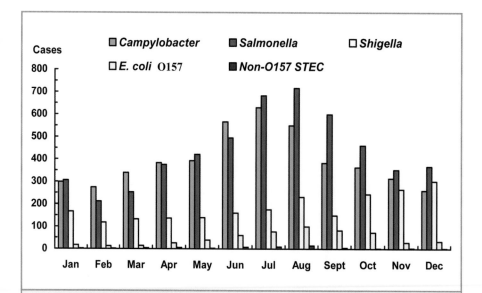

Figure 4.3 This graph illustrates how Shiga-like toxin producing *E. coli* infections occur more frequently during the warm summer months, as do other agents commonly associated with food-borne disease.

bacteria causing these infant infections were later characterized as enteropathogenic *E. coli* (EPEC). These differed from other diarrheal-associated *E. coli* strains in their mechanism of attachment to human intestinal cells.

Although EPEC used to be a major cause of outbreaks in developed countries in the 1940s and 1950s, the incidence appears to have decreased significantly.[8] Today, EPEC are better known for causing occasional, sporadic outbreaks in specific settings like hospitals and day-care centers, where highly susceptible individuals are present.

In contrast, EPEC infections continue to be a major problem in developing countries, contributing to a total of 1 million deaths per year among infants and children. EPEC infections generally occur during periods of warm, wet weather and cause severe dehydration and malnutrition in addition to diarrhea.

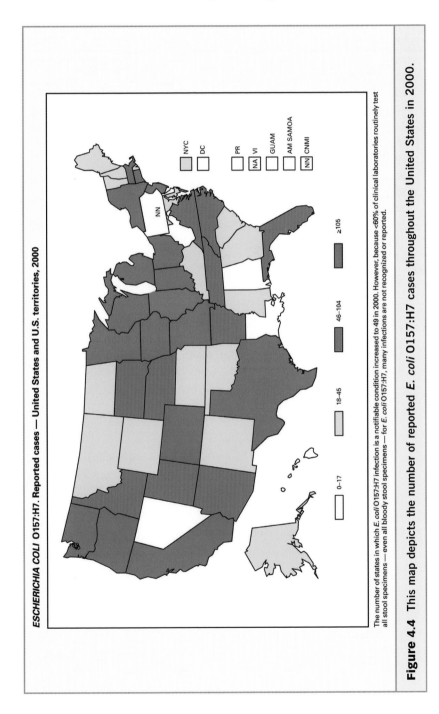

ESCHERICHIA COLI O157:H7. Reported cases — United States and U.S. territories, 2000

The number of states in which *E. coli* O157:H7 infection is a notifiable condition increased to 49 in 2000. However, because <60% of clinical laboratories routinely test all stool specimens — even all bloody stool specimens — for *E. coli* O157:H7, many infections are not recognized or reported.

Figure 4.4 This map depicts the number of reported *E. coli* O157:H7 cases throughout the United States in 2000.

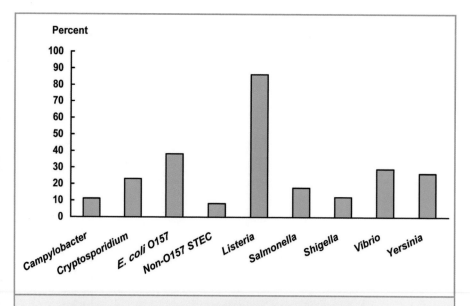

Figure 4.5 This graph shows the percentage of people who required hospitalization in 2001 because of infection with specific agents commonly associated with food-borne infections. Almost 40% of *E. coli* O157:H7 cases reported by FoodNet surveillance sites involved people who were hospitalized.

ETEC INFECTIONS

Enterotoxigenic *E. coli* (ETEC) infections are similar to EPEC infections in that they occur during the wet summer months in regions where the disease is endemic. In addition, both infections primarily target babies and children. It has been reported that approximately 20 to 60% of those visiting a region where ETEC is endemic will likely develop ETEC-associated diarrhea.[9]

EAEC AND EIEC INFECTIONS

Enteroadherent *E. coli* (EAEC) has become an increasingly common cause of diarrheal disease outbreaks in developing nations.[10] EAEC infections are associated with cases of diarrhea that last more than 14 days, and thus, these infections are often called persistent diarrhea syndrome. In Brazil, it was estimated that 68% of patients with persistent diarrhea had an EAEC infection.

Enteroinvasive *E. coli* (EIEC) infections also primarily cause sporadic outbreaks that tend to be the result of ingesting contaminated food or water. It was estimated that 5% of diarrheal disease cases among American travelers to Mexico were caused by EIEC.[11] The incidence of EIEC-associated diarrheal disease in developed nations is low, despite two large food-associated outbreaks in the United States. The first caused gastroenteritis in at least 226 people, and was spread throughout the country. The cause was serotype O124 EIEC–contaminated cheese.[12] The second outbreak, caused by serotype O143 EIEC, occurred in the early 1990s and affected 370 people in Texas. Guacamole prepared by a local caterer was identified as the source of infection.[13]

UPEC INFECTIONS

Uropathogenic *E. coli* (UPEC), which is associated with urinary tract infections, commonly affects people of all ages. The incidence of UTI in any given year is 12% among women and 3% among men. Over half of all women will have a UTI by their mid-twenties.[14] Transmission of UPEC occurs primarily by person-to-person direct contact, though fecal-oral transmission also may occur. Studies have observed a relationship between sexual activity and the development of UTI in some women. The infection is sometimes referred to as "honeymoon cystitis," since a UTI often develops in women following their honeymoon because of frequent sexual intercourse.

IMPACT OF *E. COLI* DISEASES ON THE HEALTH SYSTEM

E. coli–associated diarrheal and urinary infections are clearly a significant and costly health problem. The costs associated with UTI in otherwise healthy women were estimated at

$1.6 billion in the United States in 1995.[15] In addition, many patients in hospitals acquire a UTI or kidney infection during hospitalization for other medical conditions. This is referred to as a **nosocomial infection**. It has been estimated that nosocomial UTI infections contribute to longer hospital stays and can cost up to $451 million per year.[16]

The costs that may be attributed to *E. coli*–associated diarrheal diseases, particularly for developing countries, are currently unknown, but they are estimated to be quite significant. In the United States, all food-borne disease costs were estimated at $35 billion a year in 1997.[17] Diagnosis, medical treatment, hospitalization, and loss of paid work time for recovering or caring for a family member all contribute to the total costs that go along with these debilitating infections.

5

Clinical Diagnosis and Treatment

THE ROLE OF THE HEALTH-CARE PROVIDER

Although there are many different types of *E. coli* that can cause disease, people with *E. coli* infections often develop a few common symptoms. Most sufferers have urinary tract infections or gastrointestinal discomfort (cramping) and diarrhea. As mentioned previously, more serious diseases, such as hemorrhagic colitis and hemolytic uremic syndrome (HUS), also can result.

To prevent more serious complications from developing, health-care providers must recognize and diagnose *E. coli* infections early, particularly Shiga toxin–producing *E. coli* infections. This is important for several reasons. In the event of a food-borne outbreak of *E. coli* O157:H7, for example, rapid identification of cases enables public health officials to pinpoint and eliminate the source of infection. In addition, early disease detection allows health-care providers to utilize more effective treatment protocols.

Specimen Collection

If a provider suspects that a patient suffers from a complicated UTI or from gastrointestinal symptoms caused by *E. coli*, then he or she will most likely request a **specimen** from the patient—a sample of urine or stool that is submitted to a laboratory for testing. Generally, urine specimens are requested for UTIs, while stool specimens are obtained for gastro-intestinal problems. Following collection, the specimens are sent directly to the clinical laboratory for processing and evaluation. Unfortunately, not all hospitals and medical centers have clinical laboratories; thus, many specimens are shipped offsite to a larger **reference laboratory** that is often government-operated and provides support for hospitals and clinics that do not have the ability to evaluate specimens themselves. Offsite shipment of specimens extends the specimen processing and evaluation time. This is not ideal, particularly in cases of severe diarrheal infections caused by STEC.

Growing and Identifying *E. coli* in the Laboratory

Upon receipt in the laboratory, numerous microbiological tests

THE ROLE OF A REFERENCE LABORATORY

A reference laboratory provides support for other institutions, such as hospitals and health-care clinics, which do not have the ability or finances to evaluate laboratory specimens properly. Most states have one main laboratory that is often called the state laboratory, or state health agency, and numerous reference laboratories scattered in distinct geographic areas. These state laboratories are critical components of the public health system.

One example is the Michigan Department of Community Health Bureau of Laboratories (MDCH-BOL), housed in Lansing, Michigan. It is the fifth oldest state laboratory in the nation. It was established in 1907, when the Michigan State Board of Health appointed a bacteriologist to examine blood, sputum, urine, water, milk, and any other substance associated with disease outbreaks.

Today, the MDCH-BOL provides laboratory support for many departments within the MDCH; 49 local health departments from different regions; other state health departments in the Midwest; and hospitals and health-care providers in the state of Michigan. Additionally, MDCH-BOL works closely are performed on urine and stool specimens to determine the cause of infection. Initially, a small amount of the specimen is **subcultured**, or transferred to a growth medium for visualization and analysis. A **growth medium** is a synthetic substance that contains essential nutrients that enhance the growth of microorganisms. The medium is solidified by the addition of **agar**, which provides an ideal environment for growing bacteria. Microbiologists who suspect that E. coli is present in a stool specimen from a patient with severe diarrhea often choose **MacConkey agar** (**MAC**), whereas different media types are used to grow other bacteria (Figure 5.1).

with the CDC on outbreak investigations, research, and disease-prevention programs.

MDCH-BOL is composed of numerous sections, including microbiology—the study of microorganisms and their effects on humans. The microbiology section processes many specimens associated with bacterial infections including E. coli O157:H7-associated outbreaks and agents of bioterrorism (e.g., anthrax).

Laboratories are numbered 1 through 4, according to their biosafety level, or level of biological hazard to humans. For instance, biosafety level 1 laboratories work with microorganisms that rarely cause disease in humans (e.g., normal flora E. coli), while level 4 laboratories work with microorganisms that cause diseases that have no cure or treatment, and often lead to death. An example of an agent that requires a level 4 facility is the Ebola virus, which is considered one of the deadliest viruses that affect humans. It causes death in 50–90% of patients.[a]

a. World Health Organization. "Ebola Haemorrhagic Fever." Available online at http://www.who.int/emc/diseases/ebola/en.

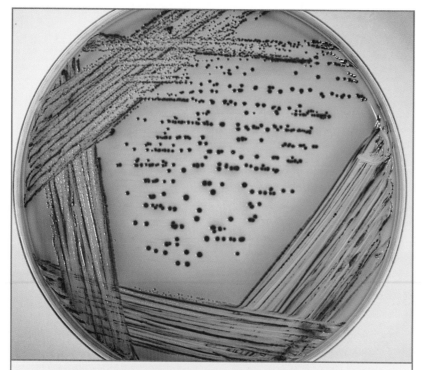

Figure 5.1 *Escherichia coli* is shown here growing on MacConkey (MAC) agar, a commonly used growth medium. *E. coli* colonies appear round, pink, and flat on MAC agar.

Trained microbiologists can identify *E. coli* "by eye" on MAC and other media, but to confirm the presence of the bacterium, more specific biochemical tests must be conducted. Biochemical characterization of bacteria is important to determine what type of bacteria is present in any given specimen. For example, **indole** is a biochemical product produced by most *E. coli*. When microbiologists perform a spot indole test on *E. coli*, the solution will turn purple. A spot indole test is useful because it is a fast, simple, and inexpensive way to rule out the presence of other harmful bacteria, such as *Salmonella* and *Shigella*. Like *E. coli*, these bacteria also cause gastrointestinal symptoms and can grow in similar environments. If microbiologists fail to perform the appropriate tests on a specimen, then an inaccurate disease diagnosis can result, which can have a negative impact on patient treatment and management.

Detecting Uropathogenic *E. coli* (UPEC)

To confirm the presence of UPEC in a urine specimen, microbiologists rely on bacterial counting. Specifically, they will count the total number of bacterial **colonies**—groups of identical organisms grown from a single parent cell—in a specified amount of urine on a MAC plate. A patient is considered to have a UTI or UPEC-associated disease if the number of bacterial colonies exceeds 100,000. In this case, microbiologists report the laboratory results directly to the health-care provider, who makes a decision regarding treatment based on colony counts, urine dipstick test results, and patient symptoms. A dipstick test, which is a quick and easy way to assess whether harmful substances are excreted in the urine, is used as an indicator to evaluate whether someone has a UTI.

Detecting Diarrhea-causing *E. coli*

Detection of the various *E. coli* types that cause diarrhea is quite difficult in a clinical laboratory. In most cases, microbiologists rely on culture-based detection methods, which involve using growth media to identify and isolate the bacteria. It is, however, extremely difficult to distinguish pathogenic from nonpathogenic *E. coli* using these methods; as a result, tests that detect bacterial characteristics (e.g., specific toxins produced by the bacteria) or genetic characteristics are considered more reliable. ETEC, for example, produces two toxins (heat-labile and heat-stable toxins) that can be detected via different laboratory techniques. Tests that detect the presence of a molecule or component specific to a microorganism (such as the heat-labile toxin) are referred to as phenotypic tests. DNA-based techniques that assess the genetic characteristics of a micro-organism (e.g., a gene sequence specific for the heat-labile toxin) are called genotypic tests. Both phenotypic (physical characteristics) and genotypic (genetic characteristics) tests are available to detect the various diarrhea-associated *E. coli* types, but many of them are expensive, tedious, and time-consuming to perform on a regular basis.

Detecting Shiga Toxin–producing *E. coli* (STEC)

Because each *E. coli* type that causes diarrheal disease relies on different mechanisms of detection, the remainder of this chapter will focus on the detection of one, STEC, which includes the O157:H7 serotype as well as other non-O157:H7 serotypes.

There are many reasons why O157:H7 STEC is difficult to detect in stool specimens. The main reason is that O157:H7 STEC cannot be identified on specific growth media, such as MAC, which is used regularly to grow *E. coli*. On MAC, STEC looks exactly like the normal *E. coli* that live in the human gut, and therefore, cannot be distinguished from other strains. Because of this, scientists have developed a new growth media called sorbitol MacConkey (SMAC) agar. It includes **sorbitol**, which enhances the detection of these bacteria. Most O157:H7 STEC strains cannot **ferment**, or utilize, sorbitol, and they appear colorless on SMAC agar, while most *E. coli* strains (which can ferment sorbitol) appear pink.

Another problem associated with O157:H7 STEC identification is that specimen processing is often not performed in a timely manner. For example, some laboratories must ship stool specimens to reference laboratories via mail for further testing. Because the specimen may be en route for up to five days, the O157:H7 STEC bacteria once present in the specimen can die or decrease to undetectable amounts. As a result, the reference laboratory may not be able to detect the bacteria in a given specimen. A similar situation would occur if a patient were treated prior to stool specimen collection.

It is important to note that identifying O157:H7 *E. coli* strains on SMAC agar does not confirm that they are STEC or, in other words, that they contain the toxin. To determine this, the laboratory must first perform other phenotypic tests besides serotyping, as well as genotypic tests.

Detecting Non-O157 STEC

Because serotypes other than O157:H7 (non-O157) can also possess the Shiga-like toxin (Stx) and are associated with severe disease, microbiology laboratories must make every effort to identify non-O157 STEC strains from stool specimens. These strains, however, are very difficult to identify using routine microbiology practices; therefore, the real frequency is likely higher than the reported frequency. In the United States, for instance, the frequency of non-O157s is not even known because most laboratories do not attempt to identify them.

Unlike O157:H7 STEC, most non-O157 STEC strains can ferment sorbitol. These strains appear pink on SMAC agar, which is how the normal *E. coli* from the human gastrointestinal tract appears. In addition, there are no definitive biochemical characteristics that can distinguish non-O157 from O157:H7 STEC. Because of the difficulties associated with detecting non-O157 STEC strains in stool specimens, microbiologists rely on both phenotypic and genotypic molecular techniques. As mentioned previously, these techniques are often time-consuming and expensive and are frequently performed only at larger reference laboratories and research institutions.

Molecular Techniques Used to Detect Both O157:H7 and Non-O157:H7 STEC

A phenotypic technique called the enzyme-linked immunosorbent assay (ELISA), which detects the presence of the Shiga-like toxin using antibodies, is becoming more popular among microbiologists. **Antibodies** are substances produced by the human immune system that specifically target harmful substances made by the bacteria. If a person is infected with STEC, the immune system will produce antibodies that bind directly to the Stx. Other immune cells will recognize this antibody-Stx complex and destroy it, thereby eliminating the infection from the person.

The ELISA technique uses a microtiter plate (Figure 5.2) with 96 wells coated with Stx-specific antibodies. In the laboratory, the stool specimen is added directly to the wells, and if Stx is present, the Stx-specific antibody will bind to it. If Stx is present, then the solution will change colors. Because the ELISA detects the presence of Stx directly, strains of all serotypes, including the non-O157 STEC, can be identified. This represents an advantage over culture-based detection methods, such as using SMAC agar, which limit detection to O157:H7 strains alone. Although ELISA is easy to use and the results are generated in just one day, it is also costly and can occasionally produce a false-positive result—that is, a result that indicates that the specimen is positive for the toxin when the toxin is not, in fact, present. Consequently, many clinical laboratories cannot afford to use ELISA regularly.

Polymerase chain reaction (**PCR**) is a genotypic test that can be used to detect STEC. PCR technology identifies whether specific DNA sequences, or genes, are present in a given laboratory specimen. When they are functioning, these genes instruct the bacterial cells to produce specific products, such as the Stx protein. In this case, the gene that encodes for Stx is called the *stx* gene (specific names of genes are italicized). Using PCR, scientists can screen for the presence of the *stx* genes in a specimen and thus determine whether a particular *E. coli* has the ability to produce Stx and cause severe disease.

Although PCR is considered a reliable and straightforward technique, it does have a few limitations. First, PCR samples are subject to contamination by other DNA sources, including DNA present on the skin of the microbiologist

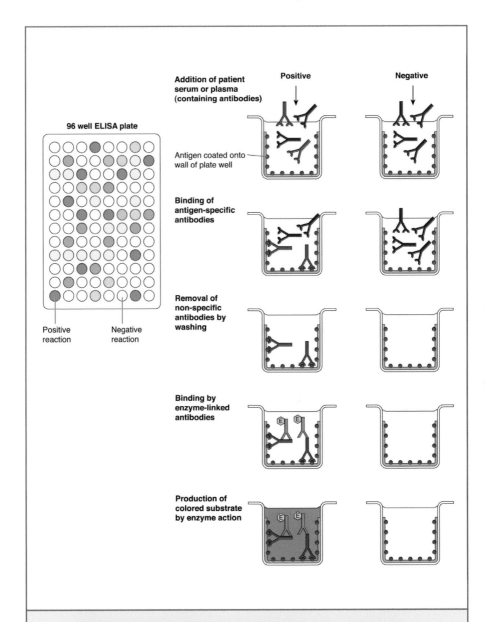

Figure 5.2 The ELISA test is used to detect the presence of Shiga toxin (Stx) and other antigens produced by microorganisms. Stx-specific antibodies bind to the antigen, which results in a detectable color change. The process of an ELISA is illustrated here.

who performs the technique. The PCR technique is also too expensive for most clinical laboratories to utilize it for routine testing.

STEC DETECTION STRATEGIES

Choosing the appropriate method to detect STEC in stool specimens depends on a number of considerations, the primary one being the expense associated with more advanced detection methods such as ELISA and PCR. Many laboratories do not use these unless a physician specifically orders them to be performed; some insurance companies do not reimburse laboratories for the costs associated with these tests, even if they may benefit the patient. This puts the laboratory in a very difficult position, since microbiologists understand the importance of conducting appropriate tests to identify the cause of specific infections. From a public health perspective, failure to perform a specific test or culture might be very serious because STEC outbreaks could potentially be missed.

Ideally, clinical laboratories should screen all stool specimens from patients suffering with severe gastrointestinal symptoms for the presence of STEC. The best techniques available today (e.g., PCR and ELISA) enable microbiologists to detect the presence of all STEC serotypes. These tests, however, should always be confirmed using standard culture-based methods and serotyping, keeping in mind that non-O157 serotypes are more difficult to find, and therefore, may require more time and patience.

Although the ELISA and PCR methods are superior to current culture-based methods for STEC detection, the proportion of clinical laboratories using these techniques is not known. A recent Michigan study found that only 52 of the 102 clinical laboratories surveyed in 2002 used SMAC agar to detect *E. coli* O157:H7 strains from bloody stool specimens. Only three laboratories used the ELISA method, and the remainder did not even culture for *E. coli*. Based on these results, it is likely that most laboratories in Michigan may have missed non-O157 STEC, and that the frequency of both O157:H7 and non-O157 STEC is underestimated.[3]

HOW ARE BACTERIAL INFECTIONS TREATED?

In 1928, our way of combating infectious diseases changed forever. That year marked the discovery of **penicillin**, the first naturally occurring antibiotic and the first to be used to treat bacterial infections in people. An **antibiotic** is a substance produced by a living organism that can kill or prevent the growth of microorganisms, including bacteria. Antibiotics work by disrupting a critical pathway in the bacterial cell cycle. Penicillin, for example, prevents the bacterium's cell wall from forming, thereby inhibiting bacterial reproduction.

Before the discovery of penicillin, death from infection was an all too common occurrence. In the early 20th century, pneumonia, tuberculosis, and diarrheal disease—all infectious diseases—were the primary causes of death in the United States, while heart disease ranked fourth. In 2001, heart disease, cancer, cerebrovascular diseases (stroke), and lower respiratory diseases ranked first through fourth, respectively, in the United States.[5] The older historical infections have decreased in frequency over time, partly due to the use of antibiotics. Today, however, although infectious diseases are no longer the main cause of death, they appear to be increasing in overall frequency. Emerging, or relatively new, diseases are contributing to the more than 170,000 deaths per year in the United States that are attributed to infectious disease.[6]

How Are *E. coli* Infections Treated?

For diarrheal diseases, health-care providers usually begin the treatment regimen by addressing the dehydration that often accompanies severe diarrheal infections. Oral rehydration therapy (ORT), which was first used to treat cholera infections,

(continued on page 66)

THE DISCOVERY OF ANTIBACTERIAL AGENTS

Ernest Duchesne, a French medical student, first discovered penicillin in 1896. Duchesne's work, demonstrating that a substance produced by a specific mold could kill bacteria, was ignored and forgotten until Alexander Fleming's rediscovery 32 years later.[a] Fleming, a Scottish physician trained as a surgeon and bacteriologist at St. Mary's Medical School in London, became interested in **antibacterial agents**— molecules or substances that can kill or prevent the growth of another organism—early in his medical career. Interestingly, his discovery of penicillin was accidental.

In the 1920s, Fleming discovered lysozyme, an enzyme that is naturally produced by the body and can be found in tears. He determined that lysozyme has an antibacterial effect, though one not strong enough to combat most infectious agents. He searched diligently for more agents until 1928. One day, Fleming was organizing his laboratory and throwing away plates containing old bacterial cultures. One plate grabbed his attention because there was a large fungus, a bread mold, growing at the top (Figure 5.3). The mold had killed all the *Staphylococcus* bacteria that were growing nearby. Fleming cultured the mold and identified it as *Penicillium notatum*, which produces an antibacterial substance referred to as penicillin.[b]

Fleming continued to work with the mold for some time, but it was difficult to grow in the laboratory. The research was taken over by Howard Florey and Ernest Chain, who continued to work on the isolation of penicillin and conducted studies documenting its antibacterial effects in mice.[c] It was not until after World War II began, however, that chemical companies started to mass-produce penicillin for use in people with bacterial infections.

In 1945, Fleming, Florey, and Chain were awarded the Nobel Prize for their work on penicillin, and one year later,

Dorothy Hodgkin, a scientist specializing in biological crystals and chemistry, determined the actual structure of penicillin. This remarkable discovery enabled the manufacture of semi-synthetic penicillins that have since been used to combat numerous bacterial infections worldwide.[d] One important example is **ampicillin**, a semi-synthetic penicillin commonly used to treat and prevent *E. coli* infections, particularly those that affect newborn babies.

a. Brown, J. C. *What the heck is penicillin?* Available online at *http://www.people.ku.edu/~jbrown/penicillin.html.*

b. WGBH Educational Foundation. *A Science Odyssey: Alexander Fleming.* 1998. Available online at *http://www.pbs.org/wgbh/aso/databank/entries/bmflem.html.*

c. Ibid.

d. Ibid.

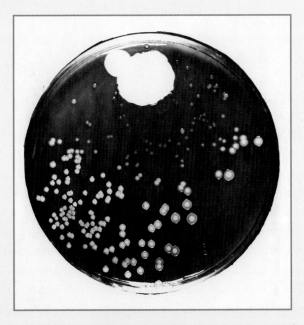

Figure 5.3 This is a photograph that Alexander Fleming himself took of an agar plate with *Staphylococcus* bacteria (small white circles) and the *Penicillium notatum* mold (top of plate).

(*continued from page 63*)

is commonly used to replace water and electrolytes lost through diarrhea. In the event that ORT fails, however, health-care professionals recommend over-the-counter drugs, such as bismuth subsalicylate (Pepto-Bismol®) and loperamide (Imodium®).

When all else fails, particularly in cases of severe and persistent bloody diarrhea, medical providers turn to antibiotics. There is considerable debate today over whether patients with STEC-associated infections or other diarrheal infections involving *E. coli* strains that produce toxins should receive antibiotics. Because the production of toxins by STEC causes most of the disease symptoms, it is unclear what effect antibiotic-induced bacterial killing has on the amount of Stx produced. Some speculate that antibiotics actually contribute to more severe disease because they kill more bacteria and the bacteria release more Stx as they die.[7] Consequently, current guidelines recommend administering antibiotics to people only if they are in the early stage of STEC disease when the bacteria are not as abundant.[8]

In contrast, antibiotics are routinely given to patients suffering from uropathogenic *E. coli* (UPEC) infections that cause both UTIs and more severe kidney complications. Health-care providers will choose antibiotics that specifically target *E. coli* that reside in the urinary tract. Newborn babies with severe *E. coli* infections (e.g., sepsis or meningitis) also are given antibiotics, which are often administered intravenously or via a shot in the arm.

Benefits of Using the Appropriate Treatments

Because diarrheal diseases contribute to so many deaths among babies and children worldwide, it is imperative to develop treatment guidelines that attempt to decrease the burden attributable to the disease. Some topics that were incorporated into recent treatment guidelines developed by the World Health Organization (WHO) include promoting rapid and effective treatments, increasing our ability to recognize key symptoms associated with severe disease, improving management of the infection at home, and educating the public regarding malnutrition risks and prevention practices (such as breastfeeding). By utilizing the appropriate methods to manage diarrheal diseases, it has been estimated that the lives of up to 1.8 million people, most of them children, could be saved each year.[9]

6

How Does *E. coli* Cause Disease?

Microorganisms contribute to disease via complex pathways that depend on multiple interactions. **Pathogenesis**, the development of disease, occurs as a result of the interactions between the host, agent, and environment. Exposure to a specific microorganism is not enough to cause disease in some individuals, though it is necessary. In the case of enterotoxigenic *E. coli* (ETEC), contaminated food or water in a certain area (environment), characteristcs of the ETEC present (agent), and the lack of an appropriate anti-ETEC immune response (host) would all interact and contribute to disease development. This chapter concentrates on a sample of host, agent, and environmental factors that are associated with *E. coli* disease pathogenesis.

WHO IS MOST AFFECTED BY *E. COLI* INFECTIONS?

To combat infectious diseases, humans must first rely on the defenses provided by their immune system. The human immune response is the result of a complex system of cells working together to eliminate a pathogen, or foreign substance, from the body. This response differs from person to person and varies in intensity, which is dependent on numerous factors, including previous exposure to a pathogen and current state of health.

OVERVIEW OF THE IMMUNE SYSTEM

Infectious agents and toxins bombard the human body regularly. In order for us to survive this constant attack, we rely on our immune system. The immune system contains three types of defense mechanisms: mechanical and chemical barriers, the innate response, and the adaptive response. The skin is the primary mechanical barrier present in humans, while chemical barriers consist of enzymes (such as lysozyme), other secreted substances, and the concentration of acid in the stomach, which is referred to as stomach pH. These all work in a nonspecific way to kill a foreign agent, or **antigen**, that enters the body.

The **innate immune response**, another nonspecific system, utilizes specialized immune cells to eliminate infectious agents or foreign substances from the body. Immune cells, such as neutrophils, basophils, eosinophils, macrophages, mast cells, and natural killer cells, are capable of destroying or eliminating antigens in the body. Before this nonspecific antigen killing occurs, however, innate immune cells must first be able to recognize foreign antigens and distinguish them from normal human cells. Specific cellular components are present on normal human cells that make this job easier. Upon recognition of a foreign antigen, innate immune cells will travel to the infection site and damage or kill the infectious agent through **phagocytosis**, the process by which the immune cells engulf and digest the antigen, or by releasing toxic chemicals into the environment (Figure 6.1).

If an antigen is contacted but cannot be eliminated by cells involved in the innate immune response, then activation of the more specific **adaptive** (or acquired) **immune response** will result, specifically targeting the antigen using specialized white blood cells. This response usually takes place 96 to 120 hours following an infection. Macrophages, for example, can bind to the foreign antigen and transport it to a **lymph node**, a mass of tissue that plays a major role in the immune response. Lymph nodes are an important part of the lymphatic system, which also includes lymph vessels, the spleen, and the thymus gland. It is similar to the cardiac system, in that immune cells move via **lymph**, a clear liquid, through the lymph vessels, just as blood cells move via blood through blood vessels. This

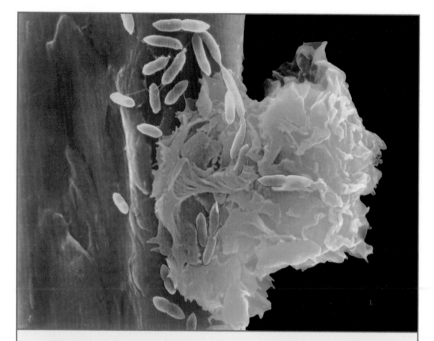

Figure 6.1 Shown here is the digestion or phagocytosis of *E. coli* bacteria (yellow) by a macrophage (pink) present on the outside of a blood vessel. This image, taken with an electron microscope, is magnified 1,315 times.

movement enables immune cells to contact foreign antigens more easily. After the macrophage-antigen complex enters the lymph node, the macrophage presents the antigen to specialized white blood cells called **T lymphocytes**. This triggers a cascade of additional immune responses. The antigen-bound T lymphocytes will signal for other T lymphocytes (cytotoxic T cells) to destroy any cells that also are presenting the recognized antigen. In addition, antigen-bound T lymphocytes stimulate the production of **B lymphocytes**, white blood cells that produce antibodies specific to the antigen. Recall that an antibody is a protein that binds to the antigen to create an antigen-antibody complex that can be recognized by the immune system and eliminated by other immune cells. These B lymphocytes will then turn into plasma cells, which are essentially factories for the production of one specific antibody type. The newly produced antibodies will patrol the body, looking for foreign antigens in the bloodstream and lymph.

The immune system is extremely complex, with each immune cell playing a specific role in the response. Interestingly, immune cells all start out as identical cells (stem cells) that differentiate into specialized immune cells (Figure 6.2). Another interesting characteristic of the immune system is that it can recognize antigens that have previously caused disease in a person. In other words, the system is capable of "remembering" which antigens or infectious agents have caused an immune response in the past. This process is performed by both T and B lymphocytes that develop into "memory" cells and continue to patrol the body for foreign invaders long after an infection has subsided. This long-term immunity can be activated from an infection or via a vaccine, the administration of an infectious agent, or component of the agent, in order to stimulate the immune response. So as not to cause the actual disease, a vaccine contains weakened or killed pathogens. The immune response is also capable of developing short-term immunity, which is usually obtained by transferring antibodies from one person to another. Newborns, for instance, acquire protective antibodies from their mothers via breastfeeding. These antibodies, however, will disappear shortly after weaning, and new antibodies will not be generated until the infant is vaccinated or gets an infection.[1]

Disease caused by most *E. coli* strains, and other infectious agents for that matter, primarily affects the very young and the very old. This is because young children and elderly people have a less effective immune response and, therefore, often have trouble fighting the infection. In addition, **immunocompromised** individuals, in whom the immune system is not functioning properly, are also at risk of developing *E. coli* infections. Exam-

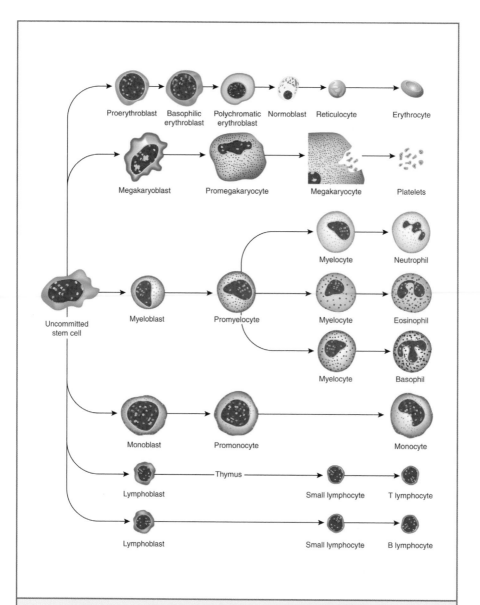

Figure 6.2 This diagram shows how human immune cells develop into cells that are capable of combating infectious pathogens and other foreign substances. Each cell begins as a stem cell and differentiates into a very specialized cell.

ples of immunocompromised individuals include people who are currently combating another serious infection, such as HIV, or those with a chronic condition, such as diabetes or cancer.

In contrast, UPEC-associated urinary tract infections (UTI) tend to affect women between 20 and 24 years of age.[2] Men of this same age group are not affected, which may be due to anatomical differences. Women have a shorter urethra, the tube-like organ used for eliminating urine, and the distance from their bowel to urethral opening is shorter, making it easier for *E. coli* to travel from the bowel, where they commonly reside, to the urinary tract.[3]

HUMAN BEHAVIORS ASSOCIATED WITH *E. COLI* INFECTIONS

Researchers speculate that specific behaviors rather than an inadequate immune response may also influence the development of *E. coli* infections. Numerous epidemiological studies have identified sexual activity as one behavior closely associated with the development of UTIs in women.

Sexual contact does not seem to be important for the development of *E. coli*–associated diarrheal infections, though person-to-person transmission does occur. In most cases, person-to-person transmission is the result of the fecal-oral route of transmission or contact with the contaminated feces of an affected individual. For example, a mother with a diarrheal infection could use the bathroom, but forget to wash her hands. Afterward, she may hug, cuddle, and feed her infant, who could subsequently develop a similar, more severe diarrheal infection a few days later. Hygiene behaviors, therefore, are extremely important, as are proper food-handling techniques.

THE PATHOGENESIS PERSPECTIVE AS VIEWED BY *E. COLI*

In order for disease to develop in any individual, an infectious agent must be able to colonize and proliferate in the host. This is not always a simple task, since the human body has a powerful immune system and is crowded with millions of microorganisms that make up our normal flora. Most infectious agents, however, have developed strategies that increase their chances of survival in this chaotic environment.

All types of *E. coli* have similar infection strategies. The first step in the disease process is to colonize the mucous membranes, while subsequently avoiding the host immune response. The *E. coli* bacteria must then multiply and compete for a larger area within the host. This proliferation and invasion of host tissues causes damage that contributes to the symptoms common to most *E. coli* infections (e.g., diarrhea).[4] Other characteristics, such as colonization factors, toxin production, pathogenesis mechanisms, the degree of **infectivity**, the **inoculum**, the **infectious dose**, and the overall virulence, differ among *E. coli* strains.

Which *E. coli* Characteristics Contribute to Disease Pathogenesis?

Because so many virulence factors have been identified in *E. coli*,

BACTERIAL VIRULENCE

The capacity of a microorganism to cause disease (its **virulence**) is measured by the severity of the resulting disease. For instance, infections caused by *E. coli* O157:H7 are usually more severe and debilitating than infections caused by ETEC, such as traveler's diarrhea. For the most part, this is because of differences in the overall virulence of the two bacterial types and can be linked to distinctions in the characteristics of each bacterium. Characteristics that enhance the virulence of any infectious agent are called **virulence factors**, and each microorganism contains a unique set of these factors that facilitate disease development.

we will only focus on the well-characterized factors that play an important role in the development of disease. This does not mean, however, that other factors are not relevant, since the development of any disease is often caused by many factors working together.

Most *E. coli* strains, including those that do not cause disease, have special structures called **fimbriae**, arm-like appendages that extend from bacteria and allow them to reach out and attach to mucous membranes. Several different types of fimbriae exist, which tend to vary by *E. coli* type. For instance, one type of UPEC fimbriae is called P pilus. This kind of fimbriae prefers to attach to the tissues that line the urinary tract.

EPEC and EHEC (e.g., *E. coli* O157:H7) produce fimbriae that attach loosely to intestinal tissues. They differ from those found on other *E. coli* types in that the fimbrial attachment phase stimulates the development of attaching and effacing lesions. These lesions represent a state of intimate adherence and are caused as the bacterium induces structural changes in the affected human tissues.[5]

Following colonization, several *E. coli* types produce potent toxins. As mentioned previously, the heat-labile and heat-stable toxins of ETEC, as well as the Shiga-like toxin of EHEC, significantly contribute to disease symptoms. These toxins are injected into human cells by the bacteria, thereby disrupting the cellular environment and facilitating the development of disease states such as diarrhea.

Avoiding the Human Immune System and Resisting Host Defenses

Lipopolysaccharide (LPS), which also is referred to as endotoxin, is part of the *E. coli* outer membrane and has demonstrated adherence capabilities in some strains. The LPS structure is quite complex and is involved in the avoidance of the human immune response as well as adherence. In particular, LPS contains some conserved regions, or parts that are found consistently in all *E. coli* strains, as well as some unique regions that make up the serotype. By changing its composition, *E. coli* can avoid recognition and elimination by the human immune system, as immune cells will not be able to recognize the new antigen.[6]

Similarly, cell invasion, which is common for EIEC strains, also enables the *E. coli* to avoid the human immune system. Instead of delivering toxins into the host cells, EIEC colonization triggers the host cell to engulf the invader and bring it inside the cell. Once inside, the bacterium remains enclosed in a protected membrane. Because this membrane is made from the host cell membrane, immune cells cannot recognize the bacterium as a foreign antigen. The protected bacterium can then move and infect adjacent cells quickly and easily (Figure 6.3).

A STATE OF CHANGE

E. coli has evolved and changed considerably over time. New outbreaks sometimes result because of changes in the virulence or pathogenic potential of old strains. If these genetic changes enhance a bacterium's survival in some way, then the bacterium will proliferate and increase in frequency relative to the other less virulent strains. This process is called **natural selection**, which is thought to have occurred in *E. coli* O157:H7 strains. Some experts speculate that a nonpathogenic *E. coli* O157:H7 strain turned into a pathogen prior to the 1982 outbreak, when it acquired the genetic components that enable it to produce the Shiga-like toxin and other virulence factors. At the same time, *E. coli* O157:H7 also acquired the ability to withstand and survive in extremely acidic environments, including foods, such as apple juice, and the stomachs of humans and cattle.[7]

RESISTING TREATMENT

In the event that a patient is suffering from an *E. coli* infection, a health-care provider often prescribes antibiotics. This is

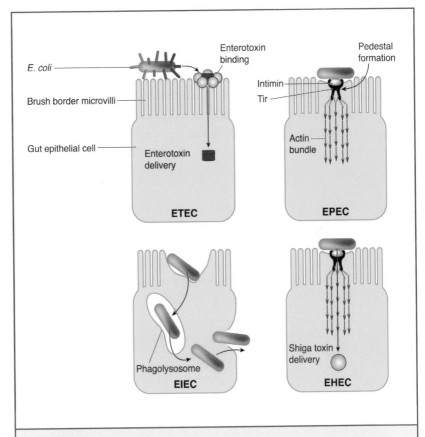

Figure 6.3 This figure demonstrates the pathogenesis of different types of *E. coli* infections. *E. coli* bacteria (in blue) are shown attaching to or invading host cells (orange). Each *E. coli* type differs in how it attaches to cells, causes changes in the host cell, produces toxins, and is able to invade cells.

particularly true for UTIs. However, *E. coli* has acquired the ability to fight back. Specifically, it has evolved mechanisms to resist or avoid being killed by antibiotics. This phenomenon, referred to as **antibiotic resistance**, has become a major public health concern worldwide. In fact, recent estimates suggest that antibiotic resistance adds an extra $100 to $200 million per year to health-care costs in the United States alone.[8]

WHY IS ANTIBIOTIC RESISTANCE SUCH A CONCERN?

If a particular infection is caused by a bacterium that is resistant to specific antibiotics, health-care providers must use alternative, or second-line, antibiotics to treat the infection. Second-line antibiotics, however, are usually more expensive and can cause more severe side effects in some people. In addition, some bacterial types, such as *Staphylococcus aureus*, are becoming resistant to second-line antibiotics (e.g., vancomycin) as well as first-line

BACTERIA FIGHT BACK: Antibiotic Resistance

A wide variety of antibiotics exist today that are commonly used to treat everything from the common cold to more severe bacterial infections (such as meningitis). Antibiotics differ with regard to their target sites, the way they kill bacteria, their concentration, and the side effects they cause. They are produced by microorganisms (e.g., *Penicillium notatum*) to kill harmful bacteria.

In order for antibiotic resistance to develop, bacteria must first come in contact with a particular antibiotic. This may occur, for example, when a health-care provider prescribes an antibiotic for a person with a suspected bacterial infection. Antibiotics do not work on viruses. So, if a patient actually has an infection caused by a virus, the antibiotic will target the bacteria found in the patient's normal flora without killing the virus.

In addition to taking antibiotics for the wrong type of infections, some patients discontinue use of a prescribed antibiotic before finishing the entire amount. In this situation, the patient will not ingest the amount necessary to kill a particular type of bacteria. This practice leads to resistance because it subjects the pathogenic bacteria as well as normal flora residents to moderate amounts of antibiotic, thereby allowing them to better tolerate the drug. Instead of being killed, newly resistant bacteria will survive the antibiotics (methicillin). If resistance to second-line antibiotics becomes widespread among *S. aureus* strains, then the infections may be virtually incurable, since no other effective alternatives are currently available.

Antibiotic Resistance in *E. coli*

UPEC strains that cause UTIs are frequently resistant to antibiotics. It is estimated that 39 to 45% of all urinary tract pathogens, most of which are caused by *E. coli*, are resistant to

course of antibiotic treatments and continue to divide and proliferate in the person long after an infection has subsided. If the same person later develops a similar infection and is treated with the same antibiotic, the resistant bacteria will be unaffected. In other words, the use of a particular antibiotic can actually help resistant bacteria by eliminating the defenseless bacteria and leaving behind the stronger, resistant strains. Overuse of antibiotics in many different settings, including health care, veterinary medicine, and agriculture, has significantly contributed to the growing problem of antibiotic resistance.

Since bacteria are constantly fighting to survive in a difficult environment, they have a unique ability to evolve or change rapidly in the face of dangers. To fight back against antibiotics, some bacteria have acquired mechanisms that facilitate resistance. For instance, some bacteria produce special enzymes that inactivate certain antibiotics, while others have developed complex systems that pump anti-biotics out of bacteria-infected cells. These mechanisms of antibiotic resistance differ by bacteria type as well as by antibiotic. Researchers have identified specific bacterial genes that are important for the development of resistance, and unfortunately, the genes can be transferred between bacteria types.

ampicillin. Resistance to another commonly used antibiotic, trimethoprim-sulfamethoxazole (TMP-SMX), ranges between 14 and 31%.[9] Individuals with a resistant *E. coli* strain are more likely to have a treatment failure, which means that the antibiotic prescribed by their health-care provider will not eliminate their infection. Therefore, another antibiotic will have to be prescribed in a second attempt to combat the infection. In some cases, **multidrug resistance**, or resistance to more than one antibiotic (such as ampicillin and TMP-SMX), occurs and can further complicate treatment. Unfortunately, people who take second-line agents, or have to take multiple antibiotics over a short period of time, often suffer longer and have more severe side effects.

Until recently, the United States has not reported antibiotic resistance among *E. coli* O157:H7 strains, though low levels of resistance have been reported in other countries. Surveillance programs conducted by the CDC have recently identified six *E. coli* O157:H7 strains isolated within the United States that were resistant to five different antibiotics. It was suggested that these multidrug-resistant strains acquired the genetic capabilities to resist antibiotics from other enteric pathogens with similar characteristics, such as *Salmonella*. In fact, in all six strains, the genes that encode the proteins involved in antibiotic resistance were found on a **plasmid**, a genetic structure that can be transferred between bacteria. This is clearly a major concern. Bacteria that share similar environments may acquire resistance readily via these transferable components, which may eventually cause a significant increase in the overall frequency of resistance.

7

Tracking *E. coli*

WHY IS TRACKING OUTBREAKS NECESSARY?

Tracking down and identifying the source or cause of an outbreak is an exciting and challenging task for an epidemiologist. In a disease outbreak situation, however, many people are affected, which occasionally causes a state of panic. Because people are concerned for their own and their family's safety, they often put pressure on public health officials, who are themselves trying to identify the outbreak cause quickly and prevent its spread. This frequently results in a very hostile environment. Despite such problems, outbreak investigations are extremely important. Not only do they enable us to control the current outbreak and prevent additional infections, but they also provide us with essential research and training opportunities and a reason to seek public, political, or legal changes (e.g., meat-processing regulations). In addition, investigations allow us to evaluate the effectiveness of current surveillance programs designed specifically to identify, control, and prevent a given disease.[1]

SURVEILLANCE SYSTEMS TO MONITOR INFECTIONS

Most outbreaks are initially discovered by health agencies that receive reports from health-care providers, clinical laboratories, citizens with knowledge of unusual cases, or established surveillance systems. This chapter will focus on the surveillance systems that public health agencies have put in place to monitor disease trends and prevent future infections.

Some surveillance systems focus on environmental settings, whereas others target hospitals or health clinics. By carefully monitoring which types of diseases or strains are present in a given environment, officials can rapidly determine whether an outbreak is in the works. Monitoring the types of microorganisms that exist in each environment is also extremely useful for identifying outbreaks. For example, continuous monitoring of *E. coli* serotypes that cause a particular disease or that are found within a certain environment helps investigators figure out whether one particular serotype has significantly increased in frequency over time.

The surveillance systems discussed in this chapter all relate to *E. coli* O157:H7, because it has a complex surveillance network that monitors multiple settings. Other systems have been designed for the other diarrhea-associated *E. coli* strains.

Surveillance of the Food Supply

The first few major *E. coli* O157:H7 outbreaks involved meat, which suggested that the bacterium was contaminating the meat supply. No one, however, understood how this contamination was occurring. Because of this, numerous studies were conducted to determine how frequently *E. coli* O157:H7 was found in processed food. Recent estimates found *E. coli* O157:H7 in up to 66 of the more than 25,000 samples of raw ground beef products tested.[2]

Surveillance Within the Agricultural Setting

After *E. coli* O157:H7 was identified in raw meat products, particularly ground beef, investigators sought to determine how the handling of livestock contributed to this contamination. For instance, it was unclear whether cattle and other livestock were asymptomatically colonized with the bacterium prior to slaughter, or whether the slaughterhouse or slaughter process was the source of the contamination.

The answers to these questions were not simple, since *E. coli* O157:H7 is quite hardy and can survive well in many environments, including cattle, slaughterhouses, and meat processed from contaminated animals or slaughterhouses. Of all types of livestock, *E. coli* O157:H7 mostly colonizes cattle and sheep, but appears to cause no symptoms in the animals. One study, for example, found that 25% of cattle shed the bacterium in their feces prior to slaughter, which implicates cattle manure as a key source of contamination. This type of contamination may explain *E. coli* O157:H7 outbreaks associated with petting farms.[3]

Some scientists speculate that *E. coli* O157:H7 can contaminate other food products via cattle manure. Many farmers use cattle manure to fertilize agricultural crops. If the manure is contaminated with the bacterium, then other foods could potentially become contaminated following exposure to the manure. This may have contributed to the 1997 alfalfa sprout outbreak in Michigan and Virginia, as well as several others.

Because the bacterium also survives well in the gastro-intestinal tract of cattle, it is often present at the time of slaughter. If a butcher accidentally nicks the intestines while preparing a carcass, then any *E. coli* O157:H7 present could potentially contaminate the entire carcass. Cattle hides often are contaminated with fecal material upon entry to a slaughter-house and, thus, may also play a role in meat contamination. The cut of meat itself has an impact on disease transmission. With meat types such as steak, only the surface becomes contaminated with bacteria; with ground meat, such as hamburger beef, the bacteria is distributed throughout the entire product during grinding. This may help explain why most meat-associated outbreaks occur with ground beef.

Surveillance of the Environment

Because *E. coli* O157:H7 can survive for weeks in water, has a low infectious dose (the amount needed to cause disease in an individual), and has caused several water-associated outbreaks in the past, surveillance systems have been established that target this source. Water sites associated with recreational activities such as swimming as well as sites that supply drink-ing water to residents are most closely monitored. Because cattle manure frequently contains *E. coli* O157:H7, runoff from agriculture fields into recreational lakes may contribute to the water contamination. Swimming pool contamination, however, is likely to result from infected people who may shed the bacterium unknowingly or, in the case of small children, via contaminated diapers.

Surveillance of Disease Cases

Hospitals and health-care clinics are excellent sites for identifying outbreaks. By evaluating diagnosis and symptom information, health-care personnel can assess whether certain diseases

WHAT ELSE CAN GO WRONG IN THE AGRICULTURAL SETTING?

Not only are cattle commonly colonized with *E. coli* O157:H7, but they also can carry antibiotic-resistant *E. coli* O157:H7 strains. One recent study found that 7.5% of sampled cattle carried *E. coli* strains that were resistant to common antibiotics. In this study, resistance was observed more frequently in the O157:H7 strains than in normal flora strains.[a]

In addition to treating human infections, antibiotics are also commonly given to farm animals or added to animal feed. Antibiotics appear to promote growth and good health among the animals, making them hardier and more eligible for sale. Consequently, millions of pounds of antibiotics are used in the agricultural setting each year,[b] which clearly has an impact on the selection of resistant strains and the subsequent transfer of them to people via the food chain.

a. Teale, C. *Veterinary Surveillance for Antimicrobial Resistance in Campylobacter, Enterococci and Other Bacteria.* Veterinary Laboratories Agency: Shrewsbury, UK 2003. Available online at *http://www.defra.gov.uk/ animalh/diseases/zoonoses/conference/amrdsstrat.htm.*

b. Shea, K. M. "Antibiotic Resistance: What Is the Impact of Agricultural Uses of Antibiotics on Children's Health?" *Pediatrics* 112 (2003): 253–258.

or symptoms are increasing in frequency. HUS caused by STEC infection, for instance, is a **notifiable disease**, which means that cases must be reported to the local health department. Local health departments are responsible for collecting the reports and submitting them electronically to the state health department, which analyzes current disease trends. Final tallies are compiled and sent to the CDC regularly. This complex reporting system is useful because it allows health agencies to have a better understanding of the disease types that are circulating in their area and to make nationwide comparisons. In addition, health agencies can determine whether these cases are a part of a larger STEC outbreak. In order to do this, epidemiologists construct epidemic curves that highlight the total number of cases by the date of symptom onset (Figure 7.1) This type of presentation can provide a clue regarding the type of transmission that is occurring in an outbreak as well.

Laboratory Surveillance

In addition to monitoring clinical diagnoses and symptoms associated with certain infections, clinical laboratories also contribute to surveillance system data. Laboratories usually monitor the types of infectious agents present in a population as well as key characteristics known to be associated with certain agents (e.g., serotype). Following identification and characterization of notifiable pathogens, such as *E. coli* O157:H7, laboratories are also required to report findings electronically using the same system described for health-care facilities. These results are tallied regularly by public health agencies. For instance, FoodNet, the national laboratory surveillance system set up to detect foodborne pathogens, identified 673 STEC infections (647 O157:H7, 26 non-O157:H7) and 44 HUS cases from certain sites in 2002. Preliminary analyses revealed that these frequencies had decreased by 8% since 1996, suggesting that prevention

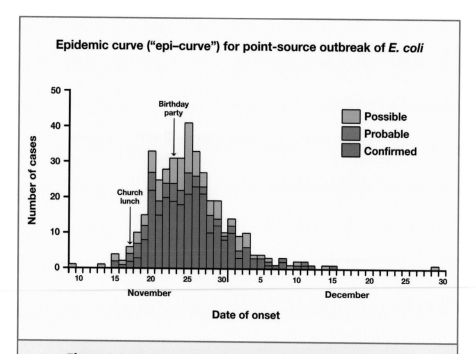

Figure 7.1 This graph shows an epidemic curve from an *E. coli* O157:H7 outbreak in 1996 involving two different events (a lunch and a birthday party). Following these events, the number of cases increased rapidly, suggesting that the people who got sick were infected at one time (referred to as a common- or point-source outbreak).

policies aimed at *E. coli* O157:H7 may be working.[4] Without laboratory surveillance systems, simple assessments of trends associated with particular infections would be difficult.

Laboratory Tools to Track
E. coli O157:H7 Outbreaks

If *E. coli* O157:H7 is identified in a patient, or from a contaminated food product, the clinical laboratory is required to perform specific molecular tests to better characterize it. Specifically, microbiologists serotype the bacterium to identify whether Shiga toxin genes are present, and use **pulsed-field gel** electrophoresis (**PFGE**) to obtain a "DNA fingerprint" of the bacterium. PFGE is a technique used to find out whether two or more **strains** of bacteria are identical. DNA is isolated from *E. coli* O157:H7 and mixed with a digestive enzyme that cuts the DNA into pieces. Sending an electrical current through the DNA on a solid medium (gel) sorts the DNA pieces by size and density. The smaller, less dense pieces will move the fastest and, thus, end up at the bottom of the gel, while the larger pieces may hardly move at all. The end result is a banding pattern that contains many lines, or DNA fragments, stacked on top of each other. Each strain has its own banding pattern, which is dependent on the number of sites available for cutting by the digestive enzyme. The resulting banding patterns are referred to as DNA fingerprints.

In the event of an outbreak, many molecular tests (serotyping, PCR, and PFGE) can be used to fully characterize the *E. coli* O157:H7 strains in question. If two strains have the

NETWORKING DNA FINGERPRINTING RESULTS: *PulseNet*

The 1993 Jack in the Box hamburger outbreak caused *E. coli* O157:H7 infection in hundreds of people. After an *E. coli* strain was isolated from either a meat or human source, scientists at the CDC performed PFGE to determine the DNA fingerprint of each strain. The results indicated that the strains found in the hamburger patties had DNA fingerprints identical to the strains from infected patients, which suggests that they came from the same source and therefore were part of the same outbreak. These results, however, were not generated in a timely manner, since PFGE takes 2 to 3 days to perform, and only a few samples can be incorporated on a gel at a time.

The thousands of samples submitted in association with this outbreak easily overwhelmed scientists at the CDC.

NETWORKING DNA FINGERPRINTING RESULTS: *PulseNet (continued)*

Because of this, officials recognized that a more efficient DNA fingerprinting system was needed to prevent future outbreaks. Therefore, they created PulseNet, a network of public health laboratories that utilize PFGE to develop DNA fingerprints of important food-borne bacteria, including *Shigella, Salmonella, E. coli* O157:H7, *Listeria monocytogenes*, and *Campylobacter*. PulseNet acts as an early warning system to detect possible food-borne outbreaks. After PFGE is completed, the DNA fingerprints are imported into an electronic database that can be shared with other laboratories nationwide. If, for example, a laboratory receives several *E. coli* O157:H7 strains over a short time period with identical DNA fingerprints, then scientists can compare those DNA fingerprints to others isolated from different regions. An increase in one particular fingerprint type in more than one geographic area might signify that an outbreak is occurring. This increase would be communicated to all public health agencies, particularly the CDC, which guides other agencies through outbreak investigations. This type of system takes the burden off of one laboratory and allows multiple laboratories to perform the testing and analyze the results simultaneously. If the PulseNet system had been in place at the time of the 1993 outbreak, it was estimated that hundreds of infections might have been prevented.[a]

Since its inception, PulseNet has been instrumental in the detection of numerous *E. coli* O157:H7 outbreaks. For instance, it was used to trace two separate outbreaks in Connecticut and Illinois that were associated with lettuce grown in California, as well as two additional outbreaks involving alfalfa sprouts in Michigan and Virginia.

a. Centers for Disease Control and Prevention. "What Is PulseNet?" 2003. Available online at *http://www.cdc.gov/pulsenet/what_is.htm*.

same Shiga toxin genes present (e.g., *stx*1 and *stx*2), but have a different PFGE banding pattern, then they are considered to be genetically different. In contrast, strains with identical gene types and PFGE banding patterns are considered identical and, therefore, may have originated from the same source. In an outbreak situation, multiple strains from multiple people may all carry strains with the same DNA fingerprint. After identifying a common fingerprint, epidemiologists and microbiologists from health agencies work together to identify a common source.

8

Perspectives on Prevention

The major *E. coli* O157:H7 outbreaks of the 1980s and early 1990s underscored the need for outbreak prevention efforts. Because *E. coli* O157:H7 is found in farm animals, meat products, and water, a complicated prevention strategy was required. Most public health officials believe that the farm represents the best site for prevention efforts because animals that are not colonized with *E. coli* O157:H7 do not run the risk of contaminating the meat or water supply. Others, however, disagree with this argument, claiming that the meat-packing industry should be responsible for preventing bacterial contamination. The issue continues to be a source of much debate.

Instead of placing the responsibility on one institution or industry, the U.S. Department of Agriculture (USDA) has adopted a farm-to-table strategy for preventing food-borne illnesses. This approach recognizes that prevention efforts will work best if individuals from different sectors of industry and society, including consumers, all work together to decrease contamination of the food supply.

PREVENTION EFFORTS FOCUSING ON THE FOOD SUPPLY

In October 1994, the USDA created an organization called the Food Safety and Inspection Service (FSIS), which is responsible for regulating and inspecting meat, poultry, and egg products to ensure that they are safe, wholesome, and correctly labeled. In 2001, FSIS inspected more than 8.2 billion poultry, 140 million heads of livestock, and 4.5 billion pounds of eggs. FSIS also monitors foreign inspection systems before allowing other countries to export meat or poultry products to the United States. Those products that are allowed to enter are always reinspected upon arrival.

For livestock, inspectors examine animals before and after slaughter to prevent any contaminated meat from being processed. Inspections are conducted randomly at more than 1,700 meat-processing plants and 100,000 retail stores distributed throughout the nation. About 250,000 other meat products, including frozen dinners, soups, sausages, and pizzas, are also inspected regularly.[1]

Prior to the creation of FSIS, federal regulations involving meat inspection were less than perfect. In fact, some refer to the old technique of bacterial detection as the "sniff-based" method, in which only foul-smelling meat products were eliminated from processing. Today, science-based procedures are used, which rely on more sensitive microbiological testing methods to identify and culture bacterial contaminants. If *E. coli* O157:H7 is detected, the DNA fingerprint will be determined by PFGE and input into PulseNet. This enables investigators to assess whether any human infections were caused by the same strain identified from the meat product. If a connection is found, FSIS will institute a meat recall.

A recall is a voluntary removal of all contaminated meat products from the market by industry in cooperation with the federal government to prevent food-borne infections. The recall process is made easier because each meat product has a date code, lot number, and, often, a store number, which enables inspectors to locate the contaminated meat rapidly. In most situations, however, this is a difficult process, since many different processing plants send meat to multiple retail stores as well as to restaurants. In April 2003, for instance, Umpqua Indian Foods of Oregon voluntarily recalled 180 pounds (82 kg) of ground beef with suspected *E. coli* O157:H7 contamination detected by FSIS inspectors. Each package of ground beef contained specific dates and lot numbers, but there was no way to track all of the meat.[2] In situations like this, FSIS relies heavily on the media and state and local health departments to inform citizens, stores, and restaurant owners of the recall and the potential health risks.

The USDA recall classification system is composed of three classes—Class I, II, and III—that differ based on the health risks to humans.[3]

> **Class I:** A health hazard situation where there is reasonable probability that the use of the recalled product will cause serious adverse health consequences or death.

> **Class II:** A health hazard situation where there is a remote probability of adverse health consequences from use of the recalled product.

> **Class III:** A situation where the use of the product will not cause adverse health consequences.

If any *E. coli* O157:H7 are detected in a meat product, then a Class I recall is generally instituted. To date, the largest recall associated with *E. coli* O157:H7 contamination occurred in 1997, when Hudson Foods Company of Arkansas recalled 25 million pounds (11.3 million kg) of frozen ground beef patties. The FSIS learned of the contaminated ground beef after several consumers got sick and reported eating the meat to the Colorado Department of Public Health and Environment.[4]

CONTAMINATION SOURCES ON THE FARM

Because cattle and other livestock are the primary source of *E. coli* O157:H7, the farm represents a good location for implementing prevention practices. However, this has proven to be very difficult, since there are numerous factors that contribute to the contamination of farm animals. In addition, colonization of cattle is usually asymptomatic and transient. This means that in order to detect the bacterium, many specimens need to be collected from the animals at multiple points in time. This tends to be both expensive and time-consuming; recent estimates suggest that 75% of dairy farm herds in the United States are colonized with *E. coli* O157:H7.[5] Though not all members of a herd are colonized, it is clearly not feasible to test every single animal in a herd.

Water troughs and feedlots, the feeding facilities used by cattle and other livestock, are also frequently contaminated. Water troughs, particularly those that are not cleaned regularly and develop sediments, provide ideal environments for the bacterium to survive, proliferate, and facilitate transmission to other animals. A recent study of 100 feedlots in 13 states found that *E. coli* O157:H7 contamination occurred in 63%.[6]

It was estimated that a member of a cattle herd often carries and sheds *E. coli* O157:H7 in its feces for up to 3 months. Some farms, however, can be contaminated for up to 2 years.[7] The duration of colonization among cattle is dependent on many factors, including diet, drinking from a contaminated water trough, age, breed type, farm conditions, temperature, *E. coli* type, immune response, and the degree of competition from normal intestinal flora.[8]

PREVENTION EFFORTS TARGETING THE AGRICULTURE INDUSTRY

Obviously, farm prevention strategies are quite complex because so many different factors contribute to colonization and contamination of cattle. Thus, numerous points of intervention have been identified that can potentially have an impact on contamination at a given farm (Table 8.1). Though

Table 8.1 Primary points of intervention that can be used at the farm to decrease the frequency of *E. coli* O157:H7 contamination

Point of intervention for *E. coli* O157:H7	Example of intervention strategy
Decrease colonization and fecal shedding frequency among cattle	1. Adding beneficial bacteria to feed to compete with *E. coli* O157:H7 or kill it. 2. Innovative vaccines containing *E. coli* O157:H7 virulence genes that stimulate an immune response in the gastrointestinal tract of cattle. 3. Bacterial viruses that kill certain bacteria (e.g., bacteriophages). 4. Farm management practices (e.g., avoid using feedlots, diet changes).
Decrease contamination in drinking water	1. Frequent cleaning (e.g., remove biofilms that trap the bacterium). 2. Remove sediments from water troughs.
Decrease contamination in manure	1. Add beneficial bacteria to kill *E. coli* O157:H7 present in farmyard. 2. Add beneficial bacteria to kill *E. coli* O157:H7 present in manure compost. 3. Adopt management practices that enable cow manure to be used only as a fertilizer for soil and not other types of produce.
Improve personal hygiene of animal handlers	1. Educate handlers about handwashing, fecal-oral transmission, and CDC guidelines. 2. Ensure that farm visitors do not contact animals and manure. Educate others about handwashing if contact occurs.

Source: Michael P. Doyle of the University of Georgia Center for Food Safety. Available online at *http://www.fsis.usda.gov.*

many researchers have implemented and evaluated prevention programs targeting farms, few have been successful at significantly decreasing the amount of *E. coli* O157:H7 contamination. A few studies that yielded positive results are highlighted here.

Eliminating *E. coli* O157:H7 Colonization in Cattle

One effort led by a University of Nebraska research team involved mixing beneficial bacteria, such as *Lactobacillus acidophilus*, into cattle feed. *L. acidophilus* is a bacteria commonly used in yogurt that has the ability to kill pathogenic bacteria such as *E. coli* O157:H7 following ingestion (Figure 8.1). The results demonstrated that the frequency of *E. coli* O157:H7 in cattle manure decreased by 61% among cattle that had eaten the enriched feed.[9]

Another study analyzed colonization frequencies among cattle fed a grain diet versus those fed a hay diet (cattle are generally fed grain). The percentage of acid-resistant *E. coli* was lower among the hay-fed cattle. Researchers suggest that hay alters the stomach acid concentration, thereby making it more difficult for some *E. coli* strains to survive.[10]

Preventing Water Contamination

A very simple intervention process, such as cleaning water troughs and removing contaminated sediments, may significantly decrease the frequency of *E. coli* O157:H7 on farms. One investigation that took place on four Wisconsin dairy farms involved sampling 15 calves for a year to identify the source of an *E. coli* O157:H7 infection. One interesting finding showed that when the drinking water troughs became contaminated with *E. coli* O157:H7, cattle that drank the water quickly began to shed the bacterium in their feces, thereby causing it to spread rapidly throughout the herd.[11]

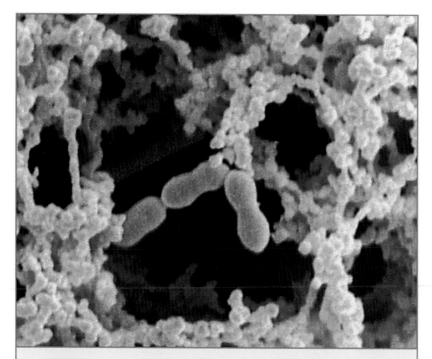

Figure 8.1 This photomicrograph shows the structure of yogurt. Different types of *Lactobacillus* bacteria (pink) are added to milk to make yogurt. When people eat them, these bacteria are beneficial because they reside in the gut and can prevent other harmful agents from invading and causing disease. Often, health-care providers advise patients to eat yogurt if they are suffering from a gastrointestinal infection or have taken antibiotics that are known to kill the normal bacteria that live in the gut.

PREVENTION EFFORTS TARGETING THE FOOD INDUSTRY AND CONSUMERS

Meat sold to retail stores is not inspected by FSIS, but rather is examined randomly by local and state inspectors. Because of this, FSIS works with a separate organization called the Association of Food and Drug Officials (AFDO), which focuses on educating retailers about food-borne disease risks. AFDO provides an educational course on meat and poultry processing at

(continued on page 99)

PREPARING MEAT FOR CONSUMPTION

Meat should always be prepared following very specific instructions. It may look fine on the outside, but it could nevertheless have been contaminated before cooking. If you are not careful, bacteria can contact other food items while you are preparing your meal, thereby promoting cross-contamination. Because of this, it is important to follow a few simple steps to keep food safe.

Before you begin to prepare meat items, you should always wash your hands with soap and water, and wash them again before eating. After cutting up and preparing meat, you can prevent contamination of other food items by scrubbing cutting boards, counter surfaces, dishes, and utensils in soapy water before reuse. Raw meat juices should never be allowed to mix with other food items. Marinades used on raw meat should be discarded and not used again on cooked meat. All meat should be cooked thoroughly; a red or pink color indicates that the meat is raw or undercooked, which means that cooking temperatures may not have been high enough to kill any bacteria that might be present. A survey conducted in 1998 found that consumers were cooking ground beef more thoroughly than they did in the past, though 16% sill served it rare or medium-rare.[a] Hamburgers, in particular, should be cooked to an internal temperature of at least 165°F (74°C). Color alone does not determine if the meat is thoroughly cooked. A meat thermometer is the best way to be sure food has reached the proper internal temperature (Figure 8.2).

a. Consumers Union of the United States, Inc. *From Moo to You.* 1999–2003. Available online at *http://www.consumerreports.org.*

PREPARING MEAT FOR CONSUMPTION *(continued)*

FOOD	°F
Ground Meat & Meat Mixtures	
Beef, Pork, Veal, Lamb	160
Turkey, Chicken	165
Fresh Beef, Veal, Lamb	
Medium Rare	145
Medium	160
Well Done	170
Poultry	
Chicken & Turkey, whole	180
Poultry breasts, roast	170
Poultry thighs, wings	180
Duck & Goose	180
Stuffing (cooked alone or in bird)	165
Fresh Pork	
Medium	160
Well Done	170
Ham	
Fresh (raw)	160
Pre-cooked (to reheat)	140
Eggs & Egg Dishes	
Eggs	Cook until yolk & white are firm
Egg dishes	160
Leftovers & Casseroles	165

Figure 8.2a To avoid food-borne illness, it is essential to cook meat and egg products thoroughly to kill *E. coli* and other bacteria that may be present. Foods must be cooked to the temperatures shown here to be sure the bacteria are killed.

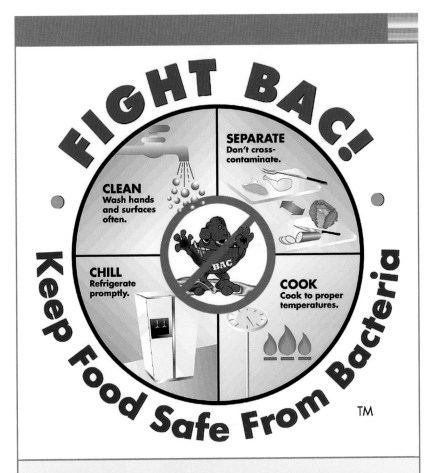

Figure 8.2b Signs like this one from the Partnership for Food Safety Education remind consumers about ways they can reduce food-borne illness. You can often obtain brochures containing this information, as well as proper cooking temperatures (see Figure 8.2a), at places where meat is sold.

(continued from page 96)

various sites around the country. The course trains individuals who regulate and inspect retail stores on the hazards associated with grinding and slicing meat, making sausage and dried meat (e.g., jerky), and the curing and smoking processes.[12]

(continued on page 102)

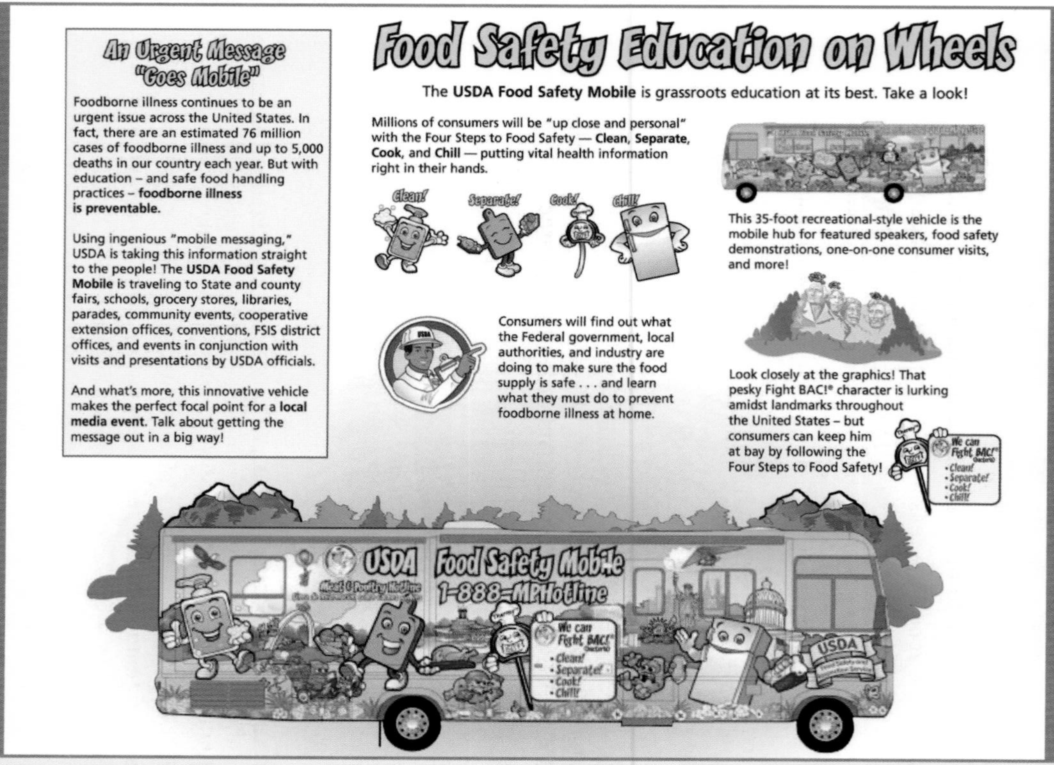

Figure 8.3 The United States Department of Agriculture (USDA) Food Safety Mobile is designed to educate consumers about food safety. It serves as a traveling headquarters for speakers, demonstrations, and information about preventing food-borne illness.

EMERGENCY SITUATIONS

A large portion of the eastern United States experienced a major power outage in August 2003 that left millions of residents without electricity for 1 to 2 days. During that time, numerous advisories were issued to residents living in certain areas to boil water before drinking and to throw out spoiled food. The reason behind these advisories was to prevent food- and water-borne infections. In Detroit, for example, the water advisories were issued because the power outage had shut down water-processing plants, which meant that sewage-contaminated water could enter the drinking water supply. In this situation, residents were told to boil water for 10 minutes and allow it to cool completely before drinking it.[a]

The food advisory was issued because bacteria can multiply rapidly in meat and poultry when the temperature rises above 40°F (4.4°C). For refrigerated and frozen foods, particularly meat, the refrigeration temperature should always be kept at or below 40°F (4.4°C), while a freezer should not fall below 0°F (-17.8°C). In the event of a power outage or other emergency, the refrigerator and freezer doors should be kept closed to maintain the appropriate temperature. Food should be thrown away if the power is out for more than 4 hours for a refrigerator or 48 hours for a freezer.

The FSIS recommends that residents always be prepared for emergency situations by having food items on hand that do not require refrigeration. When the electricity returns, frozen food can be refrozen only if the food still contains ice crystals or if the food temperature is lower than 40°F (4.4°C). When in doubt about the safety of a food item, however, it is always wise to throw it away. Warmer temperatures enable potentially harmful bacteria, such as *E. coli* O157:H7, to thrive.

a. Foodsafety.gov. "Gateway to Government Food Safety Information: Consumer Advice on Disaster Assistance." 2003. Available online at *http://www.foodsafety.gov*.

(continued from page 99)

Consumers are the best targets for prevention practices, since they are most at risk for developing a food-borne infection. Many organizations and educational programs focus on consumers. For example, the National Restaurant Association Educational Foundation's International Food Safety Council named September National Food Safety Education month, in an effort to heighten awareness about the importance of food safety. The USDA also designed the Food Safety Mobile, a colorful education and outreach vehicle that travels around the United States to teach consumers about the risks associated with mishandling food and to explain useful prevention practices for reducing the risk of food-borne illness (Figure 8.3).

9

Future Possibilities and Concerns

THE POSSIBILITIES

The past few decades have seen a major increase in research devoted to *E. coli* infections, particularly the types that contribute to diarrheal disease. Because *E. coli* O157:H7 was only discovered in 1982, there is still much to learn about the bacterium and the severe disease it causes. Many researchers as well as government agencies are devoting a significant amount of time and money to the implementation of prevention programs and innovative technologies that target *E. coli* O157:H7. These efforts are extremely important for disease eradication. This chapter will highlight some of the more important developments.

An Edible Vaccine

Administering vaccines to cattle represents a mechanism by which asymptomatic *E. coli* O157:H7 colonization can be eliminated. The traditional vaccines that are used commonly in humans to protect against many infectious diseases will not work for cattle, though some experts suggest that other types of vaccines may be effective. Edible vaccines, for instance, are currently under investigation. A recent study conducted on volunteers who agreed to eat edible potato vaccines found that the vaccine actually elicited an immune response in the individuals, enabling the development of *E. coli* antibodies (Figure 9.1). The potato vaccine is a genetically modified potato that contains genes that encode for factors

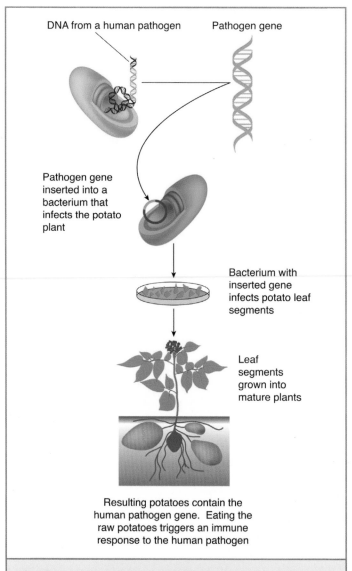

DNA from a human pathogen

Pathogen gene

Pathogen gene inserted into a bacterium that infects the potato plant

Bacterium with inserted gene infects potato leaf segments

Leaf segments grown into mature plants

Resulting potatoes contain the human pathogen gene. Eating the raw potatoes triggers an immune response to the human pathogen

Figure 9.1 This diagram illustrates how virulence genes, such as the Shiga-like toxin genes, are inserted into a bacterium that is pathogenic to plants. An infected plant incorporates the virulence genes into its DNA and produces the antigens, such as the Shiga toxin. A human immune response is triggered when a person eats the raw plant product.

(e.g., heat-labile toxin) that protect against an ETEC infection. Some speculate that the vaccination of cattle via edible vaccines may be a way to combat asymptomatic *E. coli* O157:H7 colonization, thereby preventing further spread of the bacterium through a herd.

Enhanced Detection Methods

To properly treat various *E. coli* types that cause diarrheal disease, clinical laboratories must first be able to identify the type of *E. coli* in a given specimen. Using current techniques, this is often difficult. Some researchers are now focusing on new ways to detect and isolate bacteria, such as STEC, using sophisticated molecular methods as well as simple biochemical analyses. A biochemical analysis, for instance, requires that researchers evaluate the specific biochemical profiles of all STEC strains. This will enable researchers to determine if one biochemical component could be targeted and used for detection. New growth media that distinguish among *E. coli* types also need to be evaluated. Developing better detection systems is important if scientists hope to more accurately and rapidly determine whether specific diseases are caused by STEC strains, which has serious implications for patient treatment regimens.

An Antimicrobial Spray

In August 2003, the Food and Drug Administration (FDA) announced that a Salt Lake City, Utah, company called aLF Ventures would be marketing a new product—a spray containing **lactoferrin**, a naturally occurring antimicrobial protein found in milk. The company found that spraying lactoferrin on raw beef carcasses inhibited the growth of *E. coli* and prevented the bacteria from attaching to meat surfaces. The FDA indicated that the product can be sprayed on carcasses to ward off *E. coli* O157:H7 contamination and that the substance is safe for its intended use.

THE CONCERNS

Although many investigators are currently looking into new detection and prevention methods, bacteria are constantly changing and evolving over time. Natural selection contributes to the enhancement of particular *E. coli* strains, selecting those mutations that give the bacteria an advantage in the environment—by making them unrecognizable to the human immune system, for example. There is always a possibility that currently pathogenic strains will become even more pathogenic if they acquire different virulence factors or genes that encode for antibiotic resistance. This is also true for normal flora strains. Unfortunately, a genetic change that occurs in bacteria is not an event that we can prevent or prepare for in advance.

Bioterrorism Involving the Food Supply

Recently, the U.S. federal government has invested billions of dollars to protect our nation from acts of **bioterrorism**— the use of bacteria, viruses, or the toxins produced by them as weapons. Although an act of bioterrorism is not predictable, a high level of public health preparedness can significantly affect the outcome. In January 2002, for example, the USDA received $328 million in government funding for biosecurity measures, or plans to protect the nation from the deliberate release of pathogenic biological agents, such as anthrax. Approximately $10 million of this money was allocated for the development of a food safety bioterrorism protection program. Because *E. coli* O157:H7 has a low infectious dose and causes severe disease in many people, some speculate that it could potentially be used as an agent of bioterrorism, introduced into the food supply. Though there has never been a report of this type of occurrence, this is unfortunately not a very far-fetched idea in today's world environment.

DANGEROUS SALAD

In 1981, The Dalles, an area near the Columbia River Valley in northern Oregon, gained national attention. Indian guru Bhagwan Shree Rajneesh built a large commune called the City of Rajneeshpuram on a remote ranch in the area. Hundreds of Rajneesh's followers traveled from all over the world to be a part of the cult. The local government and citizens were not very happy with their new neighbors because the cult took political control of a nearby town and had major develop-mental plans for the land in the area. This created a very hostile environment.

In September 1984, doctors in The Dalles observed a sudden increase in diarrheal disease cases caused by *Salmonella typhimurium*. Eventually, 750 people were diagnosed, all of whom had reportedly eaten food from a self-serve salad bar. Eleven different salad bars were identified and promptly shut down by the local government. After the outbreak subsided, the source of the disease remained a mystery.

Months later, the Federal Bureau of Investigation (FBI) was investigating the cult led by Bhagwan Shree Rajneesh for other activities when its agents came across a secret laboratory at the cult's commune. The laboratory contained an *S. typhimurium* strain that was genetically identical to the strains isolated at all 11 salad bars associated with the outbreak. According to news reports, cult members had introduced the bacterium into the various salad bars in an attempt to make their fellow citizens sick. Their rationale was that sick citizens would not be able to travel to the polls to vote against the cult's land-use plans.[a]

a. Eberhart-Philips, J. *Outbreak Alert*. Oakland, CA: New Harbinger Publications, Inc., 2000.

CONCLUSION

Food-borne and water-borne infections are major concerns because they pose a threat to human health and the economic growth of affected states and nations. In the United States alone, the cost associated with all food-borne disease is estimated to be at least $35 billion a year. Though the incidence of worldwide food-borne disease is difficult to measure, the World Health Organization estimated that diarrheal diseases contributed to 2.1 million deaths worldwide in 2000.[3] The various *E. coli* types that cause diarrheal disease are likely to have contributed to a large number of these deaths.

Complex prevention efforts, which rely on interaction between governments, the food industry, and consumers, are needed to eliminate the pathogens that thrive in our food and water. Unfortunately, this is not an easy task, especially with regard to *E. coli*, a ubiquitous bacterium that comes in both pathogenic and nonpathogenic varieties.

Estimates from 2003, however, suggest that the overall incidence of *E. coli* O157:H7 infections in the Untied States has decreased by 42% since 1996, with other food-borne infections demonstrating a similar decline. These data indicate that our collaborative efforts to control the pathogen may actually be working. Now, the real challenge will be to maintain the current level of control in the United States, while focusing on other nations that are disproportionately affected by *E. coli*–associated diarrheal diseases. Decreasing the rate of disease in young children, who are more susceptible to severe infections and death, is a top priority. Making these goals a reality, however, may be difficult in light of the challenges (e.g., financial, administrative, cultural) we face in trying to implement key public health practices.

Adaptive immune response—A specific immune response that is activated by the presence of an infectious agent or foreign substance (antigen) and specifically targets the antigen using specialized white blood cells (e.g., B and T lymphocytes).

Aerosol transmission—When a mist of infectious particles released from one person via coughing or sneezing is transmitted to another person.

Agar—A substance included in growth media that solidifies to provide an ideal environment for culturing and growing bacteria.

Ampicillin—The first semi-synthetic penicillin that was manufactured following the discovery of the chemical structure of penicillin.

Antibacterial agent—A molecule or substance that can kill or prevent the growth of another organism; used to treat patients with specific bacterial infections.

Antibiotic—A molecule or substance produced by a living organism that can kill or prevent the growth of another organism. Antibiotics are used to treat patients with specific bacterial infections.

Antibiotic resistance—The ability of a bacterium to develop resistance to the killing effects of certain antibiotics.

Antibodies—Proteins that are produced by specialized immune cells (B lymphocytes) that are specific for a foreign substance (antigen). An antibody helps the body eliminate infectious agents via a complex cascade of immune responses.

Antigen—A microorganism or product of a microorganism (e.g., the *E. coli* cell wall) that triggers a human immune response when recognized by specialized immune cells.

Asymptomatic colonization—A condition in which a person (host) carries a potentially harmful microorganism but experiences no disease symptoms.

Bacteriologist—Scientist who studies single-celled prokaryotic microorganisms called bacteria.

Bacterium—Single-celled prokaryotic microorganism that lacks a nuclear membrane to hold its genetic material, or DNA. Plural is *bacteria*.

Bioterrorism—The use of bacteria, viruses, or the toxins produced by these microorganisms as weapons.

Glossary

B lymphocytes—White blood cells developed in the bone marrow that are capable of producing antibodies to combat an infection. B lymphocytes play an important role in immunity to infectious diseases.

Catalyst—A protein that accelerates a reaction, but is not consumed or changed in the process.

Cell division—The separation of one cell into two cells (daughter cells).

Cell membrane—The structure that envelops a cell.

Cell wall—A complex structure located outside the cell membrane of bacteria that acts as a protective barrier. The cell wall differs among bacteria types (e.g., gram-negative versus gram-positive).

Chronic disease—Condition that is often permanent and incurable, and can leave a person permanently disabled. Chronic diseases can be both infectious and noninfectious in origin.

Colonies—Groups of identical daughter cells that originated from a single parent cell.

Colonization—The establishment of bacterial colonies within a person. Colonization may or may not lead to infection.

Commensalism—Condition when a microorganism lives on or inside a host without causing harm.

Cytoplasm—The internal contents of a cell.

Daughter cell—A cell produced from a single parent cell following cell division. A daughter cell is identical to the parent cell.

Deoxyribonucleic acid (DNA)—A double-stranded molecule that encodes the genetic information of a cell.

Diarrhea—Frequent loose or liquid stools.

Diarrheal disease—An illness in which the dominant symptom is diarrhea.

Endemic—When an infectious agent or disease is constantly present in a given population at a specific level.

Endotoxin—A substance present on the surface of gram-negative bacteria that is released when cells are destroyed by infection.

Enterohemorrhagic *E. coli* (EHEC)—*E. coli* strains that produce a potent toxin (Shiga toxin) that causes severe diarrhea and hemolytic uremic syndrome (HUS) in some people.

Epidemic—A sudden increase in the presence of an infectious agent or disease in a population. Also known as an outbreak.

Epidemiology—The study of the occurrence of disease or health-related conditions within a given population.

Eukaryote—A cell that contains a nucleus with genetic material surrounded by a defined membrane, as well as other important cellular structures.

Facultative anaerobe—A microorganism that can survive either with or without oxygen.

Fecal-oral route—Transmission of infectious agents via ingestion of food or water that has been contaminated by feces.

Ferment—When specific microorganisms oxidize or utilize compounds.

Fimbriae—Rigid arm-like appendages that extend from the bacterial cell surface and facilitate attachment to and colonization of human mucous membranes via adherence factors. Fimbriae are common to most *E. coli* strains.

Flagella—Tail-like appendages on cells that are responsible for locomotion but not attachment. Singular is *flagellum*.

Food-borne disease—An infection or illness caused by a microorganism that was present in food or water.

Fungus—A group of flowerless and seedless plants (e.g., molds, mushrooms, and yeast) that are asexual and reproduce via spores.

Gastroenteritis—Inflammation of the stomach and intestinal lining that causes nausea, diarrhea, stomach pain, and weakness. Many different infectious agents, including various *E. coli* types, cause gastroenteritis.

Gastrointestinal (GI) tract—Organ structures that include the oral cavity, esophagus, stomach, intestines, rectum, and anus.

Genes—Structures located in the chromosomal material of cells that contain hereditary information that is transferred between cells and people.

Glossary

Genitourinary tract—The organs and structures that include the kidneys, ureters, bladder, and urethra.

Gram-negative—Refers to the type of bacteria that cannot retain color of the initial stain during the Gram stain procedure. Gram-negative organisms are often found in the gastrointestinal tract of humans.

Gram-positive—Refers to the type of bacteria that retain the color of the initial stain during the Gram stain procedure.

Growth medium—A synthetic substance that contains essential nutrients that enhance the growth of microorganisms for culture in a laboratory.

Hemolytic uremic syndrome (HUS)—A rare condition that most often affects young children and may lead to kidney failure.

Host—An organism that is infected or colonized with a microorganism.

Immunocompromised—When a person's immune system is not functioning properly, thereby making the individual more susceptible to infections.

Incidence—The rate at which a disease or infectious agent spreads among people in a given population during a specific time period.

Indole—A biochemical product that is formed following degradation of tryptophan present in a solution. *E. coli* can produce indole, and can be identified based on this biochemical characteristic.

Infectious disease—A disease caused by infection with an agent such as a virus, bacterium, or parasite.

Infectious dose—The amount of infectious agent required to cause disease in an individual.

Infectivity—An infectious agent's ability to cause disease in a susceptible individual.

Innate immune response—A nonspecific immune response that uses specific immune cells (e.g., macrophages and natural killer cells) to eliminate infectious agents or foreign substances (antigens) from the body.

Inoculum—The amount of infectious agent present in a given substance (e.g., food or water). Plural is *inocula*. Larger inocula are more likely to contribute to disease symptoms.

Lactoferrin—A protein found in milk that has antimicrobial properties.

Lipopolysaccharides (**LPS**)—Polysaccharides that contain lipids (fats) that act as endotoxins in bacteria. They extend out of the bacterial cell wall of gram-negative bacteria (e.g., *E. coli*) and consist of three parts that determine the bacterial serotype.

Lymph—A clear fluid that carries immune cells throughout the lymphatic system, which comprises the lymph vessels, lymph nodes, thymus, and spleen.

Lymph node—A mass of tissue that is part of the lymphatic system and plays a role in the immune response. Lymph nodes are the sites where B and T lymphocytes mature.

MacConkey agar (**MAC**)—A specific type of growth medium used to identify *E. coli*, which appear flat, round, and pink.

Multicellular—Refers to organisms (such as humans) that are composed of many types of cells.

Multidrug resistance—The condition when a microorganism is able to withstand the killing effects of several antibiotic types.

Mutation—An alteration or change in the genetic material of a cell.

Natural selection—Process by which the strongest organisms survive diseases and other challenges, and then produce offspring that have the traits that enabled the original organisms to survive.

Normal flora—The millions of microorganisms that normally reside in the human body. They produce essential vitamins and help protect humans from invasion by disease-causing microorganisms; however, in some cases, they can become pathogens.

Nosocomial infection—An infection acquired in a hospital setting.

Notifiable disease—Disease or infectious agent that must be reported to a health department or governmental official.

Nucleotides—The building blocks of DNA.

Nucleus—The major organelle of eukaryotic cells that contains the chromosomes, or genetic material, within an envelope.

Glossary

Opportunistic infections—Infections caused by a microorganism that does not normally cause disease, but only does so in certain situations (e.g., in immunocompromised people).

Outer membrane—Part of the bacterial cell wall that is composed of proteins and lipopolysaccharides.

Pandemic—An epidemic that occurs in multiple countries within a particular period of time.

Parasite—An organism (e.g., *Giardia lamblia*) that obtains food and shelter from another organism (e.g., a human), causing harm or being of no advantage to the host organism.

Pathogen—A disease-causing organism.

Pathogenesis—The development of a disease.

Penicillin—The first naturally occurring antibiotic discovered, as well as the first used to treat bacterial infections in humans.

Phagocytosis—The process by which immune cells, such as macrophages, engulf and digest infectious agents or foreign substances (antigens).

Phospholipid—A type of lipid found in all living cells and in the bilayers of cell membranes.

Plasmid—A small independent piece of chromosomal DNA that is capable of making copies of itself and has the ability to transfer between bacteria.

Polymerase chain reaction (PCR)—A molecular technique that enables researchers to assess whether specific DNA sequences (e.g., those specific to *E. coli* toxin genes) are present in a laboratory specimen.

Polysaccharide—A chain of simple sugar molecules (monosaccharides) that are present in the capsule region of bacteria.

Prevalence—The number of people in a population who have a specific disease or infectious agent divided by the total number of people in the population.

Prokaryote—A unicellular microorganism that has genetic material flowing freely inside the cell rather than enclosed within a nucleus.

Pulsed-field gel electrophoresis (PFGE)—A molecular technique that creates a unique DNA fingerprint, or banding pattern, for each bacterial strain tested. The technique is useful for investigating outbreaks.

Reference laboratory—A government-operated laboratory that provides support for other institutions, such as hospitals and health-care clinics, that do not have the ability or finances to evaluate laboratory specimens properly.

Reservoir—An organism (e.g., human) or environment (e.g., water) that harbors a pathogenic infectious agent that can be transmitted to other organisms.

Risk factors—Types of behavior, exposure, or inherited characteristics that are associated with the development of a particular disease or acquisition of a particular infectious agent. Risk factors are identified based on epidemiological evidence and they vary by organism and disease.

Serotype—The form of polysaccharide capsule present in bacteria. Serotyping is a tool used to distinguish between bacterial strains.

Shiga toxin—A potent toxin produced by enterohemorrhagic *E. coli* (EHEC) that is released into intestinal tissues and contributes to severe diarrhea and other complications in humans.

Sorbitol—A type of sugar that is used in growth media to detect the presence of some bacterial types (e.g., *E. coli* O157:H7).

Specimen—A sample (e.g., blood or urine) taken from a diseased individual that is submitted to a laboratory for testing.

Sporadic—Refers to a disease or infectious agent that occurs randomly in an isolated manner and is not endemic or epidemic.

Strain—A specific group with its own characteristics.

Subculture—To transfer cells, such as bacteria, to a solid medium (e.g., growth medium with agar) so that they can be visualized and analyzed.

Surveillance system—A network relying on the interactions of numerous people that is used to monitor or survey the occurrence of disease or infectious agents in a given population.

T lymphocytes—White blood cells developed in the thymus that circulate throughout the body to detect infectious agents or foreign substances (antigens). T lymphocytes play a critical role in the immune response and elimination of antigens.

Glossary

Unicellular—Refers to a microorganism that comprises only one cell (e.g., a bacterium).

Uropathogenic *E. coli* (UPEC)—A type of *E. coli* that commonly causes urinary tract infections or pyelonephritis, a severe kidney infection.

Vaccine—A preparation containing a weakened or dead infectious agent that is used to stimulate the immune system to produce antibodies. Stimulation of the immune response will lead to immunity, or resistance to future infections by the same agent.

Vector—An indirect transmission mode in which a person can become infected with an infectious agent via another organism (e.g., a mosquito).

Virulence—The capacity of an organism to produce disease after infection.

Virulence factors—Characteristics of infectious agents that facilitate the development and enhance the virulence of disease (e.g., Shiga toxin).

Virus—Intracellular parasite that relies on a host for replication and survival. Viruses are composed of either RNA or DNA, and a protein coat.

CHAPTER 2

1. Smith, H. R., and T. Cheasty. "Diarrhoeal Diseases due to *Escherichia coli* and *Aeromonas*." *Topley and Wilson's Microbiology and Microbial Infections*, eds. L. Collier, A. Balows, and M. Sussman. London: Oxford University Press, 1998.

CHAPTER 3

1. McGinn, A. P. "The Resurgence of Infectious Diseases." *Epidemic! The World of Infectious Disease*, ed. R. DeSalle. New York: The New Press, 1999.

2. World Health Organization. "World Health Report, December 2003." Available online at *http://www.who.int/entity/whr/2003/en/Facts_and_Figures_en.pdf*.

3. Watts, S. *Epidemics and History: Disease, Power and Imperialism*. New Haven, CT: Yale University Press, 1997.

4. Rosen, G. *A History of Public Health*. Baltimore: Johns Hopkins University Press, 1993.

5. Baqui, A. H., R. E. Black, R. B. Sack, et al. "Epidemiological and Clinical Characteristics of Acute and Persistent Diarrhea in Rural Bangladeshi Children." *Acta Paediatrica* 381 (Suppl.) (1992): 15–21.

6. Murray, C., and A. Lopez. *Global Health Statistics, Vol. 2*. World Health Organization, World Bank, and Harvard School of Public Health, 1996.

7. World Health Organization. "World Health Report, December 2003."

8. McGinn, 1999.

9. Claeson, M., and M. H. Merson. "Global Progress in the Control of Diarrheal Diseases." *Pediatric Infectious Disease Journal* 9 (1990): 345–355.

10. Black, R. E. "Diarrheal Diseases." *Infectious Disease Epidemiology: Theory and Practice*, eds. K. E. Nelson, C. M. Williams, and N.M.H. Graham. Gaithersburg, MD: Aspen Publishers, Inc., 2001.

11. Black, R. E., K. H. Brown, et al. "Longitudinal Studies of Infectious Diseases and Physical Growth of Children in Rural Bangladesh. II. Incidence of Diarrhea and Association with Known Pathogens." *American Journal of Epidemiology* 115 (1982): 315–324.

12. Bateman, M., and C. McGahey. "A Framework for Action: Child Diarrhea Prevention." *Global Healthlink* (September 9, 2001).

13. Abbasi, K. "The World Bank and World Health: Healthcare Strategy." *British Medical Journal* 318 (1999): 933–936.

14. Claeson, M., and M. H. Merson. "Global progress in the control of diarrheal diseases." *Pediatric Infectious Disease Journal* 9 (1990): 344–355.

15. Adam, A. "Biology of Colon Bacillus Dyspepsia and its Relation to Pathogenesis and to Intoxication." *Jahrb Kinderberth* 101 (1923): 295.

16. Kauffmann, F. "The Serology of the coli Group." *Journal of Immunology* 57 (1947): 71–100.

17. Ørskov I., I. K. Wachsmuth, et al. "Two New *Escherichia coli* O groups: O172 from Shiga-like Toxin II-Producing Strains (EHEC) and O173 from Enteroinvasive *E. coli* (EIEC)." *Acta Pathologica et Microbiologica Scandinavica* 99 (1991): 30–32.

18. Centers for Disease Control and Prevention, National Center for Infectious Diseases, Traveler's Health. *Safe Food and Water*. 2003. Available online at *http://www.cdc.gov/travel/foodwater.htm*.

Notes

19. Smith, H. R., and T. Cheasty. "Diarrhoeal Diseases due to *Escherichia coli* and *Aeromonas*." *Topley and Wilson's Microbiology and Microbial Infections*, eds. L. Collier, A. Balows, and M. Sussman. London: Oxford University Press, 1998.

CHAPTER 4

1. Fenner, F., A. J. Hall, and W. R. Dowdle. "What is eradication?" *The Eradication of Infectious Diseases*, eds. W. R. Dowdle and D. R. Hopkins. West Sussex, England: John Wiley, 1998.

2. Black, R. E. "Diarrheal Diseases." *Infectious Disease Epidemiology: Theory and Practice*, eds. K. E. Nelson, C. M. Williams, and N.M.H. Graham. Gaithersburg, MD: Aspen Publishers, Inc., 2001.

3. Griffin, P. M., and R. V. Tauxe. "The Epidemiology of Infections Caused by *Escherichia coli* O157:H7, Other Enterohemorrhagic *E. coli* and the Associated Hemolytic Uremic Syndrome." *Epidemiologic Reviews* 13 (1991): 60–98.

4. Mead, P. S., and P. M. Griffin. "*Escherichia coli* O157:H7." *Lancet* 352 (1998): 1207–1212.

5. Centers for Disease Control and Prevention. "Summary of Notifiable Diseases—United States, 2000." *Morbidity and Mortality Weekly Report* 49 (2002): 1–102. Available online at *http://www.cdc.gov*.

6. Bray, J. "Isolation of Antigenically Homogeneous Strains of *Bact. coli neapolitanum* from Summer Diarrhea in Infants." *Journal of Pathology and Bacteriology* 57 (1945): 239–247.

7. Giles, C., and G. Sangster. "An Outbreak of Infantile Gastro-enteritis in Aberdeen. The Association of a Special Type of *Bact. coli* with the Infection."
Journal of Hygiene 46 (1948): 1–9; Smith, J. "The Association of Certain Types (alpha and beta) of *Bact. coli* with Infantile Gastroenteritis." *Journal of Hygiene* 47 (1949): 221–226.

8. Nataro, J. P., and J. B. Kaper. "Diarrheagenic *Escherichia coli*." *Clinical Microbiology Reviews* 11 (1998): 142–201.

9. Ibid.

10. Ibid.

11. Wanger, A. R, B. E. Murray, P. Echeverria, et al. "Enteroinvasive *Escherichia coli* in travelers with diarrhea." *Journal of Infectious Diseases* 158 (1988): 640–642.

12. Tulloch, A. R., K. J. Ryan, S. B. Formal, et al. "Invasive Enteropathic *Escherichia coli* Dysentery." *Annals of Internal Medicine* 79 (1973): 13–17.

13. Gordillo, M. E., G. R. Reeve, J. Pappas, et al. "Molecular Characterization of Strains of Enteroinvasive *Escherichia coli* O143, Including Isolates from a Large Outbreak in Houston, Texas." *Journal of Clinical Microbiology* 30 (1992): 889–893.

14. Foxman, B., R. Barlow, H. d'Arcy, et al. "Urinary Tract Infection: Estimated Incidence and Associated Costs." *Annals of Epidemiology* 10 (2000): 509–515.

15. Ibid.

16. Jarvis, W. R. "Selected Aspects of the Socioeconomic Impact of Nosocomial Infections: Morbidity, Mortality, Cost, and Prevention." *Infection Control and Hospital Epidemiology* 17 (1996): 552–557; Saint, S. "Clinical and Economic Consequences of Nosocomial Catheter-Related Bacteriuria." *American Journal of Infection Control* 28 (2000): 68–75.

17. World Health Organization. *Food safety and foodborne illness: Fact sheet N237*. World Health Organization, 2002. Available online at *http://www.who.int/mediacentre/factsheets/fs237/en/*.

CHAPTER 5

1. Paton, J. C., and A. W. Paton. "Methods for Detection of STEC in Humans." *Methods in Molecular Medicine: E. coli: Shiga Toxin Methods and Protocols*, eds. D. Philpott and F. Ebel. Totowa, NJ: Humana Press, Inc., 2003.

2. March, S. B., and S. Ratnam. "Sorbitol-MacConkey Medium for Detection of *Escherichia coli* O157:H7 Associated with Hemorrhagic Colitis." *Journal of Clinical Microbiology* 23 (1986): 869–872.

3. Dyke, J. Personal communication. (2003).

4. Eberhart-Philips, J. *Outbreak Alert*. Oakland, CA: New Harbinger Publications, Inc., 2000.

5. United States National Center for Health Statistics. National Vital Statistics Report, Vol. 51 (5), March 14, 2003. Available online at *http://www.cdc.giv.nchs*.

6. Gannon, J. C. *The Global Infectious Disease Threat and its Implications for the United States*. National Intelligence Council, 2000. Available online at *http://www.cia.gov/cia/reports/nie/report/nie99-17d.html*.

7. Mead, P. S., and P. M. Griffin. "*Escherichia coli* O157:H7." *Lancet* 352 (1998): 1207–1212.

8. Paton and Paton, 2003.

9. World Health Organization (WHO). *Reducing Mortality from Major Killers of Children*. 2003. Available online at *http://www.who.int/inf-fs/en/fact178.html*.

CHAPTER 7

1. Centers for Disease Control and Prevention. *EXCITE: Epidemiology in the Classroom*. National Center for Chronic Disease Prevention and Health Promotion, 2002. Available online at *http://www.cdc.gov/excite/classroom/outbreak_objectives.htm*.

2. Food Safety and Inspection Service. *Microbiological Results of Raw Ground Beef Products Analyzed for Escherichia coli O157:H7 Calendar Year 2003*. United States Department of Agriculture, 2003. Available online at *http://www.fsis.usda.gov/OPHS/ecoltest/ecpositives.htm*.

3. Elder, R. O., J. F. Keen, G. R. Siragusa, et al. "Correlation of Enterohemorrhagic *Escherichia coli* O157:H7 Prevalence in Feces, Hides, and Carcasses of Beef Cattle During Processing." *Proceedings of the National Academy of Sciences USA* 97 (2000): 2999–3003.

4. Centers for Disease Control and Prevention. "Preliminary FoodNet data on the incidence of foodborne illnesses—Selected sites, United States, 2002". *Morbidity and Mortality Weekly Report* 53 (16) (2003): 338. Available online at *http://www.cdc.gov*.

CHAPTER 8

1. United States Department of Agriculture. "Food Safety." *Agriculture Fact Book*. Washington, D.C.: U.S. Government Printing Office, 2002. Available online at *http://www.usda.gov*.

2. Food Safety and Inspection Service Recall Release. "Oregon Firm Recalls Ground Beef Products for Possible *E. coli* O157:H7." 2003. Available online at *http://www.fsis.usda.gov/OA/recalls/prelease/pr021-2003.htm*.

Notes

3. Food Safety and Inspection Service. "FSIS Food Recalls." 2002. Available online at *http://www.fsis.usda.gov/OA/background/bkrecalls.htm.*

4. Food Safety and Inspection Service. "Hudson Foods Recalls Beef Burgers Nationwide for *E. coli* O157:H7." 1997. Available online at *http://www.fsis.usda.gov/oa/recalls/prelease/pr015-97.htm.*

5. Hancock, D. D., T. E. Besser, D. H. Rice, et al. "Longitudinal Study of *Escherichia coli* O157:H7 in Fourteen Cattle Herds." *Epidemiology and Infection* 118 (1997): 193–195.

6. Dargatz, D. A., S. J. Wells, L. A. Thomas, et al. "Factors Associated with the Presence of *Escherichia coli* O157:H7 in Feces of Feedlot Cattle." *Journal of Food Protection* 60 (1997): 466–470.

7. Mechie, S. C., P. A. Chapman, and C. A. Siddons. "A Fifteen-Month Study of *Escherichia coli* O157:H7 in a Dairy Herd." *Epidemiology and Infection* 118 (1997): 17–25.

8. Sanchez, S., M. D. Lee, B. G. Harmon, et al. "Animal Issues Associated with *Escherichia coli* O157:H7." *Journal of the American Veterinary Medical Association* 221 (2002): 1122–1126.

9. Miller, V. "Good Bacteria Look Promising for Reducing *E. coli.*" *Research Nebraska.* Lincoln, NE: University of Nebraska-Lincoln Agricultural Research Division, 2002. Available online at *http://ard.unl.edu/rn/0902/ecoli.html.*

10. Diez-Gonzalez, F., T. R. Callaway, M. G. Kizoulis, et al. "The Role of Grain Feeding in the Dissemination of Acid-Resistant *Escherichia coli* from Cattle." Agricultural Research Service, 1998. Available online at *http://warp.nal.usda.gov.*

11. Gallep, G. "Hunting Down a Dangerous Intruder." *Science Report.* University of Wisconsin-Madison College of Agricultural and Life Sciences, 1998.

12. Food Safety and Inspection Service. Office of Policy, Program Development, and Evaluation. "Farm-to-Table Food Safety." Available online at *http://www.fsis.usda.gov.*

Abbasi, K. "The World Bank and World Health: Healthcare Strategy." *British Medical Journal* 318 (1999): 933–936.

Adam, A. "Biology of Colon Bacillus Dyspepsia and its Relation to Pathogenesis and to Intoxication." *Jahrb Kinderberth* 101 (1923): 295.

Baqui, A. H., R. E. Black, R. B. Sack, et al. "Epidemiological and Clinical Characteristics of Acute and Persistent Diarrhea in Rural Bangladeshi Children." *Acta Paediatrica* 381 (Suppl.) (1992): 15–21.

Bateman, M., and C. McGahey. "A Framework for Action: Child Diarrhea Prevention." *Global Healthlink* (September 9, 2001).

Black, R. E. "Diarrheal Diseases." *Infectious Disease Epidemiology: Theory and Practice*, eds. K. E. Nelson, C. M. Williams, and N.M.H. Graham. Gaithersburg, MD: Aspen Publishers, Inc., 2001.

Black, R. E., K. H. Brown, et al. "Longitudinal Studies of Infectious Diseases and Physical Growth of Children in Rural Bangladesh. II. Incidence of Diarrhea and Association with Known Pathogens." *American Journal of Epidemiology* 115 (1982): 315–324.

Bray, J. "Isolation of Antigenically Homogeneous Strains of *Bact. coli neapolitanum* from Summer Diarrhoea in Infants." *Journal of Pathology and Bacteriology* 57 (1945): 239–247.

Brown, J. C. *What the heck is penicillin?* 2001. Available online at *http://www.people.ku.edu/~jbrown/penicillin.html.*

Centers for Disease Control and Prevention. *EXCITE: Epidemiology in the Classroom.* National Center for Chronic Disease Prevention and Health Promotion, 2002. Available online at *http://www.cdc.gov/excite/classroom/outbreak_objectives.htm.*

———. "Preliminary FoodNet data on the incidence of foodborne illnesses—Selected sites, United States, 2002." *Morbidity and Mortality Weekly Report* 52 (15) (2003): 340–343.

———. "Summary of Notifiable Diseases—United States, 2000." *Morbidity and Mortality Weekly Report* 49 (2002): 1–102.

———. *What Is PulseNet?* 2003. Available online at *http://www.cdc.gov/pulsenet/what_is.htm.*

Centers for Disease Control and Prevention, National Center for Infectious Diseases. *Traveler's Health: Safe Food and Water,* 2003. Available online at *http://www.cdc.gov/travel/foodwater.htm.*

Bibliography

Claeson, M., and M. H. Merson. "Global Progress in the Control of Diarrheal Diseases." *Pediatric Infectious Disease Journal* 9 (1990): 345–355.

Consumers Union of the United States, Inc. *From Moo to You.* 1999–2003. Available online at *http://www.consumerreports.org*.

Dargatz, D. A., S. J. Wells, L. A. Thomas, et al. "Factors Associated with the Presence of *Escherichia coli* O157:H7 in Feces of Feedlot Cattle." *Journal of Food Protection* 60 (1997): 466–470.

Diez-Gonzalez, F., T. R. Callaway, M. G. Kizoulis, et al. "The Role of Grain Feeding in the Dissemination of Acid-Resistant *Escherichia coli* from Cattle." Agricultural Research Service, 1998. Available online at *http://warp.nal.usda.gov*.

Dyke, J. Personal communication, 2003.

Eberhart-Philips, J. *Outbreak Alert.* Oakland, CA: New Harbinger Publications, Inc., 2000.

Elder, R. O., J. F. Keen, G. R. Siragusa, et al. "Correlation of Enterohemorrhagic *Escherichia coli* O157:H7 Prevalence in Feces, Hides, and Carcasses of Beef Cattle During Processing." *Proceedings of the National Academy of Sciences USA* 97 (2000): 2999–3003.

Fang, G. D., A. A. M. Lima, C. V. Martins, et al. "Etiology and Epidemiology of Persistent Diarrhea in Northeastern Brazil: A Hospital-Based, Prospective, Case-Control Study." *Journal of Pediatric Gastroenterology and Nutrition* 21 (1995): 137–144.

Fenner, F., A. J. Hall, and W. R. Dowdle. "What is eradication?" *The Eradication of Infectious Diseases*, eds. W. R. Dowdle and D. R. Hopkins. West Sussex, England: John Wiley, 1998.

Food and Drug Administration. FDA News. "Lactoferrin Considered Safe to Fight *E. coli.*" 2003. Available online at *http://www.fda.gov*.

Food Safety and Inspection Service. "Biosecurity and the Food Supply." 2002. Available online at *http://www.fsis.usda.gov/OA/background/biosecurity.htm*.

———. "FSIS Food Recalls." 2002. Available online at *http://www.fsis.usda.gov/OA/background/bkrecalls.htm*.

———. "Hudson Foods Recalls Beef Burgers Nationwide for *E. coli* O157:H7." 1997. Available online at *http://www.fsis.usda.gov/oa/recalls/prelease/pr015-97.htm*.

———. *Microbiological Results of Raw Ground Beef Products Analyzed for Escherichia coli O157:H7 Calendar Year 2003.* United States Department of Agriculture, 2003. Available online at *http://www.fsis.usda.gov/OPHS/ecoltest/ecpositives.htm.*

———. Office of Policy, Program Development, and Evaluation. "Farm-to-Table Food Safety." Available online at *http://www.fsis.usda.gov/oppde/fslgrs/farm.htm.*

———. Recall Release. "Oregon Firm Recalls Ground Beef Products for Possible *E. coli* O157:H7." 2003. Available online at *http://www.fsis.usda.gov/OA/recalls/prelease/pr021-2003.htm.*

Foxman, B., and P. Brown. "Epidemiology of Urinary Tract Infections: Transmission and Risk Factors, Incidence, and Costs." *Infectious Disease Clinics of North America* 17 (2003): 227–241.

Foxman, B., R. Barlow, H. d'Arcy, et al. "Urinary Tract Infection: Estimated Incidence and Associated Costs." *Annals of Epidemiology* 10 (2000): 509–515.

Foxman, B., S. D. Manning, P. Tallman, et al. "Uropathogenic *Escherichia coli* Are More Likely than Commensal *E. coli* To Be Shared Between Heterosexual Sex Partners." *American Journal of Epidemiology* 156 (2002): 1133–1140.

Gallep, G. "Hunting Down a Dangerous Intruder." *Science Report.* University of Wisconsin-Madison College of Agricultural and Life Sciences, 1998.

Gannon, J. C. *The Global Infectious Disease Threat and its Implications for the United States.* National Intelligence Council, 2000. Available online at *http://www.cia.gov/cia/reports/nie/report/nie99-17d.html.*

Gateway to Government Food Safety Information. "Consumer Advice on Disaster Assistance." 2003. Available online at *http://www.foodsafety.gov/~fsg/fsgdisas.html.*

Gibbons, N. E., and R. G. E. Murray. "Proposals Concerning the Higher Taxa of Bacteria." *International Journal of Systemic Bacteriology* 28 (1978): 1–6.

Giles, C., and G. Sangster. "An Outbreak of Infantile Gastroenteritis in Aberdeen. The Association of a Special Type of *Bact. coli* with the Infection." *Journal of Hygiene* 46 (1948): 1–9.

Gordillo, M. E., G. R. Reeve, J. Pappas, et al. "Molecular Characterization of Strains of Enteroinvasive *Escherichia coli* O143, Including Isolates from a Large Outbreak in Houston, Texas." *Journal of Clinical Microbiology* 30 (1992): 889–893.

Bibliography

Graunt, J. *Natural and Political Observations Made upon the Bills of Mortality: London, 1662.* Baltimore, MD: Johns Hopkins University Press, 1939.

Green, E. "The Bug that Ate the Burger." *Los Angeles Times,* June 6, 2001.

Griffin, P. M., and R. V. Tauxe. "The Epidemiology of Infections Caused by *Escherichia coli* O157:H7, Other Enterohemorrhagic *E. coli* and the Associated Hemolytic Uremic Syndrome." *Epidemiologic Reviews* 13 (1991): 60–98.

Hancock, D. D., T. E. Besser, D. H. Rice, et al. "Longitudinal Study of *Escherichia coli* O157:H7 in Fourteen Cattle Herds." *Epidemiology and Infection* 118 (1997): 193–195.

Hennekens, C. H., and J. E. Buring. *Epidemiology in Medicine.* Boston/ Toronto: Little Brown, 1987.

Hippocrates. "On Airs, Waters, and Places." *Medical Classics,* Vol. 3, 1938.

Hooten, T. M., A. E. Stapleton, P. Roberts, et al. "Perineal Anatomy and Urine-Voiding Characteristics of Young Men and Women with and without Recurrent Urinary Tract Infections." *Clinical Infectious Diseases* 29 (1999): 1600–1601.

Jarvis, W. R. "Selected Aspects of the Socioeconomic Impact of Nosocomial Infections: Morbidity, Mortality, Cost, and Prevention." *Infection Control and Hospital Epidemiology* 17 (1996): 552–557.

Kauffmann, F. "The Serology of the coli Group." *Journal of Immunology* 57 (1947): 71–100.

March, S. B., and S. Ratnam. "Sorbitol-MacConkey Medium for Detection of *Escherichia coli* O157:H7 Associated with Hemorrhagic Colitis." *Journal of Clinical Microbiology* 23 (1986): 869–872.

Mazzulli, T. "Resistance Trends in Urinary Tract Pathogens and Impact on Management." *Journal of Urology* 168 (2002): 1720–1722.

McGinn, A. P. "The Resurgence of Infectious Diseases." *Epidemic! The World of Infectious Disease,* ed. R. DeSalle. New York, NY: The New Press, 1999.

Mead, P. S., and P. M. Griffin. "*Escherichia coli* O157:H7." *Lancet* 352 (1998): 1207–1212.

Mechie, S. C., P. A. Chapman, and C. A. Siddons. "A Fifteen-Month Study of *Escherichia coli* O157:H7 in a Dairy Herd." *Epidemiology and Infection* 118 (1997): 17–25.

Miller, V. "Good Bacteria Look Promising for Reducing *E. coli.*" *Research Nebraska.* Lincoln, NE: University of Nebraska-Lincoln, 2002.

Moon, H. W., S. C. Whipp, R. A. Argenzio, et al. "Attaching and Effacing Activities of Rabbit and Human Enteropathogenic *Escherichia coli* in Pig and Rabbit Intestines." *Infection and Immunity* 41 (1983).

Murray, C., and A. Lopez. *Global Health Statistics, Vol. 2.* World Health Organization, World Bank, and Harvard School of Public Health, 1996.

Murray, R.G.E. *Fine Structure and Taxonomy of Bacteria, Microbial Classification.* Cambridge, MA: Cambridge University Press, 1962.

Nataro, J. P., and J. B. Kaper. "Diarrheagenic *Escherichia coli.*" *Clinical Microbiology Reviews* 11 (1998): 142–201.

Ørskov I., I. K. Wachsmuth, et al. "Two New *Escherichia coli* O groups: O172 from Shiga-like Toxin II-Producing Strains (EHEC) and O173 from Enteroinvasive *E. coli* (EIEC)." *Acta pathologica et microbiologica Scandinavica* 99 (1991): 30–32.

Paton, J. C., and A. W. Paton. "Methods for Detection of STEC in Humans." *Methods in Molecular Medicine: E. coli: Shiga Toxin Methods and Protocols,* eds. D Philpott and F. Ebel. Totowa, NJ: Humana Press, Inc., 2003.

Paustian, T. University of Wisconsin-Madison, 2003. Available online at *http:// www.bact.wisc.edu/MicrotextBook/BacterialStructure/MoreCellWall.html.*

Ramel, G. Earth-Life Web Productions, 2003. Available online at *http://www.earthlife.net/cells.html.*

Riley, L. W., R. S. Remis, S. D. Helgerson, et al. "Hemorrhagic colitis associated with a rare *Escherichia coli* serotype." *New England Journal of Medicine* 308 (1983): 681–685.

Rosen, G. *A History of Public Health.* Baltimore, MD: Johns Hopkins University Press, 1993.

Saint, S. "Clinical and Economic Consequences of Nosocomial Catheter-Related Bacteriuria." *American Journal of Infection Control* 28 (2000): 68–75.

Sanchez, S., M. D. Lee, B. G. Harmon, et al. "Animal Issues Associated with *Escherichia coli* O157:H7." *Journal of the American Veterinary Medical Association* 221 (2002): 1122–1126.

Schindler, L., D. Kerrigan, and J. Kelly. *Science Behind the News: Understanding the Immune System.* National Cancer Institute, 2003. Available online at *http://press2.nci.nih.gov/sciencebehind/immune/immune08.htm.*

Bibliography

Shea, K. M. "Antibiotic Resistance: What Is the Impact of Agricultural Uses of Antibiotics on Children's Health?" *Pediatrics* 112 (2003): 253–258.

Smith, H. R., and T. Cheasty. "Diarrhoeal Diseases due to *Escherichia coli* and *Aeromonas.*" *Topley and Wilson's Microbiology and Microbial Infections,* eds. L. Collier, A. Balows, and M. Sussman. London, England: Oxford University Press, 1998.

Smith, J. "The Association of Certain Types (alpha and beta) of *Bact. coli* with Infantile Gastroenteritis." *Journal of Hygiene* 47 (1949): 221–226.

Soper, G. A. "The Curious Case of Typhoid Mary." *Academic Medicine: Journal of the Association of American Medical Colleges* 15 (1939): 698–712.

Stanier, R. Y., and C. B. van Niel. "The Main Outlines of Bacterial Classification." *Journal of Bacteriology* 42 (1941): 437–466.

Teale, C. *Veterinary Surveillance for Antimicrobial Resistance in Campylobacter, Enterococci and Other Bacteria.* Veterinary Laboratories Agency Shrewsbury, 2003. Available online at *http://www.defra.gov.uk/animalh/diseases/zoonoses/conference/ctealeppt.htm.*

Tulloch, A. R., K. J. Ryan, S. B. Formal, et al. "Invasive enteropathic *Escherichia coli* dysentery." *Annals of Internal Medicine* 79 (1973): 13–17.

United States Department of Agriculture. "Food Safety." *Agriculture Fact Book.* Washington, D.C.: U.S. Government Printing Office, 2002. Available online at *http://www.usda.gov.*

United States Department of Health and Human Services, Centers for Disease Control and Prevention, Office of Communication, Division of Media Relations. 2003. Available online at *http://www.cdc.gov/od/oc/media/pressrel/r030717a.htm.*

United States National Center for Health Statistics. National Vital Statistics Report, Vol. 51 (5), March 14, 2003. Available online at *http://www.cdc.giv.nchs.*

University of Arizona. "Prokaryotes, Eukaryotes, & Viruses Tutorial." *The Biology Project,* 1999. Available online at *http://www.biology.arizona.edu/cell_bio/tutorials/pev/page1.html.*

Van Voris, B. "Jack in the Box ends *E. coli* suits." *The National Law Journal.* November 17, 1997.

Wanger, A. R., B. E. Murray, P. Echeverria, et al. "Enteroinvasive *Escherichia coli* in travelers with diarrhea." *Journal of Infectious Diseases* 158 (1988): 640–642.

Watanabe, Y., K. Ozasa, J. H. Mermin, et al. "Factory Outbreak of *Escherichia coli* O157:H7 Infection in Japan." *Emerging Infectious Diseases* 5 (1999): 424–428.

Watts, S. *Epidemics and History: Disease, Power and Imperialism.* New Haven, CT: Yale University Press, 1997.

WGBH Educational Foundation. *A Science Odyssey: Alexander Fleming.* 1998. Available online at *http://www.pbs.org/wgbh/aso/databank/entries/bmflem.html.*

———. *A Science Odyssey: Fleming Discovers Penicillin.* 1998. Available online at *http://www.pbs.org/wgbh/aso/databank/entries/dm28pe.html.*

Whittam, T. S., E. A. McGraw, and S. D. Reid. "Pathogenic *Escherichia coli* O157:H7: A model for Emerging Infectious Diseases." *Emerging Infections: Biomedical Research Reports,* ed. R. M. Krause. New York, NY: Academic Press, 1998.

World Health Organization. *Food safety and foodborne illness: Fact sheet N237.* World Health Organization, 2002. Available online at *http://www.who.int/mediacentre/factsheets/fs237/en/.*

———. *Reducing Mortality from Major Killers of Children.* 2003. Available online at *http://www.who.int/mediacentre/factsheets/fs178/en/.*

Websites

Cells Alive!
www.cellsalive.com

Cellular Biology
www.biology.arizona.edu/cellbio/tutorials/pev/page1.html

Centers for Disease Control and Prevention (CDC)
www.cdc.gov/

E. coli Index
http://web.bham.ac.uk/bcm4ght6/res.html

EXCITE: An Introduction to Epidemiology
www.cdc.gov/excite/classroom/intro_epi.htm

EXCITE: How to Investigate an Outbreak
www.cdc.gov/excite/classroom/outbreak.htm

National Food Safety Education Month
Partnership for Food Safety Education
www.foodsafety.gov/~fsg/september.html

Overview of Infectious Diseases, United States
Central Intelligence Agency (CIA)
www.cia.gov/cia/reports/nie/report/nie99-17d.html

PulseNet, Centers for Disease Control and Prevention (CDC)
www.cdc.gov/pulsenet/what_is.htm

Summary of Notifiable Diseases,
Centers for Disease Control and Prevention (CDC)
www.cdc.gov/mmwr/preview/mmwrhtml/mm4953a1.htm

Understanding the Immune System, National Cancer Institute
http://press2.nci.nih.gov/sciencebehind/immune/immune00.htm

United States Department of Agriculture,
Food Safety and Inspection Service
www.fsis.usda.gov/

World Health Organization (WHO)
www.who.int

Index

Index

Index

Picture Credits

17: Lambda Science Artwork
19: © Dr. David Phillips/Visuals Unlimited
20: © Gladden Willis, M.D./Visuals Unlimited
21: Lambda Science Artwork
22: © Dr. Dennis Kunkel/Visuals Unlimited
26: Information from World Health Organization (WHO)
33: Source: US National Center for Health Statistics, *National Vital Statistics Report*, vol. 51, no. 5.
44: National Geographic Society
47: The FoodNet Surveillance Report, 2001
48: The FoodNet Surveillance Report, 2001
49: *MMWR*, Vol. 49, no. 53.

50: The FoodNet Surveillance Report, 2001
56: © Gladden Willis/Visuals Unlimited
61: Lambda Science Artwork
65: © Bettmann/CORBIS
70: © Dr. Dennis Kunkel/Visuals Unlimited
72: Lambda Science Artwork
77: Lambda Science Artwork
86: Source: CDC
96: © SIMKO/Visuals Unlimited
99: Courtesy of the Partnership for Food Safety Education
100: Courtesy of the Partnership for Food Safety Education
104: Lambda Science Artwork

Cover: © Dr. Fred Hossler/Visuals Unlimited

About the Author

Shannon Manning grew up in Northville, Michigan. She obtained a B.S. in Biology at the University of Michigan, Ann Arbor in 1993. Afterwards she pursued a MPH in hospital and molecular epidemiology with a concentration in public health genetics, and a Ph.D. in epidemiologic science at the University of Michigan School of Public Health. Dr. Manning worked on various research projects involving uropathogenic *E. coli* and group B *Streptococcus*, and completed her graduate work in 2001. In 2002, she was awarded an emerging infectious diseases (EID) research fellowship through the Centers for Disease Control and Prevention (CDC) and the Association of Public Health Laboratories (APHL) where she was placed at the Michigan Department of Community Health, Bureau of Laboratories in Lansing, Michigan. Her primary research projects focused on shiga-like toxin producing *E. coli* (e.g., *E. coli* O157:H7) and *Neisseria meningitidis*.

Following completion of her fellowship in September 2004, Dr. Manning will be employed as an Assistant Professor at Michigan State University (MSU) in the Departments of Food Safety and Toxicology, and Pediatrics and Human Development. At MSU, she will continue to work on research projects involving shiga-like toxin producing *E. coli* and group B *Streptococcus*. She currently lives in Howell, Michigan with her husband and two young sons.

About the Editor

The late I. Edward Alcamo was a Distinguished Teaching Professor of Microbiology at the State University of New York at Farmingdale. Alcamo studied biology at Iona College in New York and earned his M.S. and Ph.D. degrees in microbiology at St. John's University, also in New York. He had taught at Farmingdale for over 30 years. In 2000, Alcamo won the Carski Award for Distinguished Teaching in Microbiology, the highest honor for microbiology teachers in the United States. He was a member of the American Society for Microbiology, the National Association of Biology Teachers, and the American Medical Writers Association. Alcamo authored numerous books on the subjects of microbiology, AIDS, and DNA technology as well as the award-winning textbook *Fundamentals of Microbiology*, now in its sixth edition.